The Compass Book of 30 Day Challenges Vol.1

The 30-day compass longevity challenge for living a healthier and longer life

Dr. Chio Ugochukwu

Copyright©2024 Dr. Chio Ugochukwu

Published by Bundant Enterprises
3053 Rancho Vista Blvd H-197
Palmdale , CA 93551

ISBN: 9798335954242

Printed in the United States of America

Disclaimer

The information contained in this book is based on research and the personal and professional experience of the author. It is solely for informational and educational purposes and should not be regarded as a substitute for professional, legal, tax, psychological or medical advice. Any attempt to diagnose or treat an illness should be done under the care of a healthcare professional. The author and publisher do not advocate any healthcare protocol but believe the information in this book should be available to the public. Ideas on ways people can get more peace and happiness in their relationships and their lives are shared in this book. The author assumes no liability or responsibility for any adverse effects or consequences from the use of any information, idea or instruction contained in this book.

Dedication

The Compass book of 30-day challenges consists of many volumes of books that are dedicated to improving self-mastery, better health, and becoming better versions of ourselves. This Compass book of 30-day challenges vol.1, is the 30-day compass longevity challenge for those who want to live a healthier, longer and better life through simple steps and holistic habits. Are you ready to begin your own 30-day longevity challenge for living a healthier and longer life today?

Table of Content

"Desire is the key to motivation.
But it's determination and commitment to an unrelenting pursuit of your goal....A commitment to excellence...that will enable you to attain the success you seek."

Mario Andretti

Introduction

You will learn how to live a healthier, more positive, less stressful, and longer life as you get older if you make a commitment to do the daily challenges in this 30-day compass longevity challenge for living a healthier and longer life. This book is the first volume in the compass book of 30-day challenges.

After many years of trying different ways of helping myself and others improve their health and wellness and live a healthier, happier and longer life, I found out doing 30-day challenges is one of the best ways to hold yourself accountable and help you form the purpose-driven holistic habits that will help you achieve specific goals and improve specific aspects of your life one step and one day at a time.

Over the years, I have used different 30-day compass challenges to become better at managing daily stress, maintaining a healthy weight, and becoming better at taking care of yourself through more consistent self-care and the challenges that will help you develop holistic habits and simple steps to live a healthier, longer and better life. Do you want to stay healthy, active, independent, and live a more fulfilled life as you get older, or do you want to spend your time unintentionally going from one clinic and hospital to another being treated for one illness or another?

If you want to be able to hang out with your friends, go on vacations, participate in your friends' milestones or your kids and grandkids milestones like graduations, birthdays, weddings and other festivals and events that you enjoy doing as you get older then read this book to learn about how you can use the 30-day compass longevity challenge to help you live a healthier and longer life

You will also learn practical and easy ways to make adjustments that will help you improve your self-care and increase your peace of mind and joy of living as you get older. You will learn how to live the telomeric lifestyle!

Did you know that the first key to living longer after 50 is consistency in your daily exercise and physical activity? Don't live in denial or form the habit of always having reasons or excuses for not doing your daily exercise. Don't forget that with the help of the compass profile and the compass method the transformation that you need is within your power.

You can use the 8 keys to longevity and the compass method as the basis for doing this 30-day compass longevity challenge, which is the first volume or vol 1, in this Compass Book of 30-day challenges.

Begin by writing down your challenge type and doing your self-evaluation in the next few pages. This is the compass 30-day longevity challenge!

——30 DAY CHALLENGE——

CHALLENGE TYPE

NOTES

Check or mark beach day of the challenge that you have done.

12 COMPASS LONGEVITY GUIDELINES

Do you?	1	2	3	4	5	6	7	8	9	10
Meditate on 3 things you are grateful for every day										
Do 10,000 steps daily										
Sleep At Least 7 hours A Day										
Eat 50g of fiber daily										
Do daily self-accountability										
Effectively manage daily stress										
Lower daily expectations										
Maintain a healthy weight										
Keep your appointments and yearly physical										
Have Supportive relationships										
Eat five servings of vegetables and fruit daily										
Write 3 good things that happened to you every day										

Before you go further in this Compass 30-day challenge for longevity, begin by doing a self-evaluation on how consistently you use or follow the 12 compass longevity guidelines for living a healthier and longer life. Mark X on the number that represents how frequently you consistently carry out the compass longevity guidelines in your daily life.

A score of 1 means that you are either not practicing the guideline at all in your daily life or that you hardly follow each guideline. A score of 10 for each guideline shows that you consistently practice or make use of the guidelines every day. If the total score of the numbers you have marked for each guideline is 12, it shows that you are very inconsistent in putting the guidelines into daily practice. A total score of 120 will show that you consistently follow the guidelines every day without fail and are doing an excellent job. Your total score will likely be between 48 and 72 and will show the guidelines you need to work on. Do another self-evaluation at the end of the 30-day challenge to find out how you improved.

Day 1: Begin your 10,000 steps per day challenge today

Begin your 30-day longevity challenge by going for 10,000 steps a day. If you have been mostly sedentary and haven't done much walking begin with 20 minutes of walking or 2,000 steps per day. If you already do 6,000 steps every day, challenge. yourself to add another 2,000 steps today. If you already do 10,000 steps a day or about 100 minutes of walking a day, challenge yourself to add another 2,000 steps per day. Research and studies indicate that increasing your physical activity can help you live longer.

If you don't know how many steps you take every day, do your own 72-hour walking audit to determine how many steps you take on average every day. Write down how many steps you walk every day for 3 days, then get the average to know how many steps you walk every day. Don't forget that in this 30-day compass longevity challenge, starting is more important than delaying or procrastinating.

Why is daily walking important?

Research has shown that people as old as 69 years and above who exercise regularly have the heart, lung, and muscle fitness of healthy people as young as 30 years and younger (Crouch, 2019). Walking is one of the easiest ways you can exercise regularly. Wouldn't you like to feel much younger than your age as you get older?

Here are a few things you need to do on DAY 1, as part of your 30-day challenge for longevity:

*Walk with what you have or get some comfortable walking shoes. If you are going to do most of your walking inside the house, you can walk barefoot.

 *Walk 10,000 steps today if you are already used to walking , if not begin with 2,000 steps today or about 20 minutes of walking today.

*Write down how many minutes of exercise you did on day 1. Did you do 15 minutes, 30 minutes, 45 minutes or 60 minutes of you did today?

Do you know that according to the National Institute of Health, only about 30 percent of people between 45 years and 64 years engage in leisure-time physical activity, and for those 65 years above the percentage drops to 15 percent and less (NIH News, 2017). According to the AARP, only about 17 % of Americans 50 years and above, do at least 150 minutes of exercise every week.

What is the integrative link between exercise and physical activity and antiaging and living longer? **It is the telomere or specific-DNA structures found at both ends of the chromosomes in our cells.**

According to Bringham Young University researchers, exercise has antiaging effects at the cellular level because increasing physical activity increased the length of telomeres at the end of chromosomes which are usually shorter with age. The study also found that those who exercise had a "biological age" that was about nine years younger(Baines, 2020; Crouch 2019). Why does increasing the length of telomeres in cells have such a positive impact on longevity?

Research shows that those with shorter telomeres have a poorer survival or shorter lifespan, due to an increase in mortality from heart and infectious diseases.

Why is telomere length important? Telomere length is sometimes seen as a biological clock that can be used to determine the lifespan of a cell and an organism (Shammas,2011).

*Do you know that there are many lifestyle changes or factors that can affect the length of a telomere?

Lack of exercise is one of the lifestyle factors that can significantly shorten your

---

telomere length and could reduce your longevity.

*Write down how many hours you spent sitting down today?

Therefore, if you choose to spend most of your time sitting down without exercise, you are choosing a less telomeric lifestyle.

Research also shows that telomere length is more in active people than inactive people, irrespective of whether the exercise was vigorous or moderate.

How many minutes did you spend exercising or staying physically active today? Write it down.

Remember that 10 minutes of walking is about 1,000 steps. Since on average people have 2 to 2.5 feet per step, it takes about 2,000 steps to cover a mile. This means that 10,000 steps per day is equal to 100 minutes of exercise every day and about 5 miles of walking every day.

While the main goal of day 1 of the 30 day longevity challenge is to get you to walk at least 10,000 steps every day, starting from day 1, one way can get to its equivalent of 100 minutes of daily physical activity is to combine the steps from your formal physical activity period with the steps you take during activities like doing your chores, walking from one meeting to another, gardening or during other outdoor activities, to find out the total number of minutes, steps or miles, you have done in a day

You should attempt to exercise at least four or five times a week for 45 minutes or more per period. You can include walking or something simple like doing jump ropes and push-ups.

An important integrative link is learning how physical activity affects your cellular and vascular health. As you already know, consistent physical activity helps to increase the length of your telomeres at the cellular level by helping to decrease the rate of shortening of telomeres that occur with age.

What is the impact of exercise at the vascular level? Exercise protects the endothelium or cells lining the vessels by reducing reactive oxygen species and reducing inflammation and increases the cellular metabolic state by affecting your increasing mitochondria (Sorriento, Vaia and Iaccarino, 2021).

Mitochondria are critical to human health and in organs in which damaged mitochondria accumulate more organ damage or disorders occur(Sorriento, Vaia and Iaccarino, 2021).

The integrative strategy here is to think of your mitochondria anytime you exercise or feel like not exercising. You can compare mitochondria to the energy source in your house or the batteries in your computers or smart phones or devices. No matter how expensive your phone is or how well the circuit in your computer is you cannot do much with it, when the battery is not working, or the energy source is unreliable or malfunctioning. When the mitochondria or energy packets in your cells malfunction, a lot can go wrong in your mind, body and spirit.

Whenever possible, you should take the stairs instead of the elevator, as little things like that will do wonders for your body. Research has shown that if you started exercising between 40 and 60 years of age, you would reduce your risk of having stroke that can significantly reduce your chances of living longer. This shows that it is really never too late to start exercising or form the habit of consistently increasing the level of your physical activity.

Do not think that it is either you are getting everything right or everything is wrong. If you plan to walk 60 minutes a day but due to circumstances beyond your control you were able to do only 25 minutes, you have not failed. Do the 25 minutes that day, then do 95 minutes the next day to make it up. This still makes a total of 120 minutes in two days. On the third day you can go back to 60 minutes a day. Be flexible.

Make sure you keep track of your progress. Get a guide to aging well journal or workbook to help you keep track of your progress. How many steps do you take every day? If you really become good at it , you can do 50 pushups a day. Remember that the goal is to make the exercise as tolerable as you can for yourself. You can simply stick to 20 push-ups a day, ten in the morning then ten in the evening. Track your habit of exercising regularly.

In the following Habit Tracker to 12, represent the habits you are tracking and 1 to 31, represent the days. the following habits with the habit tracker:

If you do the activities labelled 1 to 12, on day1, day2 or other days from 1 to 30, mark it with an X in the box, to track your habit.

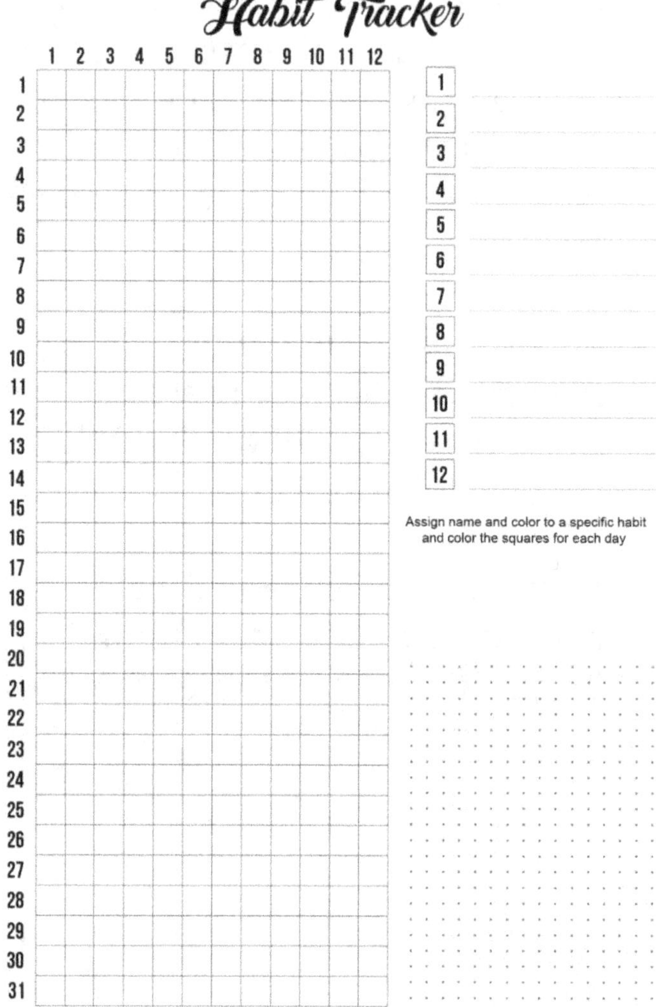

Habit Tracker
1 2 3 4 5 6 7 8 9 10 11 12
1
2
3
4
5
6
7
8
9
10
11
12
Assign name and color to a specific habit
and color the squares for each day

Track the following habits with the habit tracker:

1 Walk 10,000 steps every day

2 Do 20 pushups every day

3 Do 300 jump rope reps every two days

4 Give yourself a positive self-talk every day

5 Drink one glass of water before every meal

6 Measure your blood pressure once a week

7 Sleep at least 7 hours a day

8 Take your supplements daily

9 Eat 5 servings of fruits and vegetables everyday

10 Eat 50g of fiber every day

11 Do your daily self-care activities

12 Keep your daily Compass Stress Index
to 0 or 1 per week

Day 2: Get more consistency in physical activity by cutting down on key distractions

Challenge yourself on day 2 to get more consistency in your daily physical activity. This means you have to build on what you did on day 1. If you got to 10,000 steps on day, do it again on day2 by cutting down further on distractions. If you were so distracted or too tired to get to 10,000 steps on day1, try again on day2.

*What are the distractions stopping you from being consistent with your daily physical activity?

What distracted you?

Was it watching TV?

Was it talking on the phone?

Was it playing too much on your phone or device or computer?

Was it always putting off, when you would actually begin to walk?

Was it a negative encounter or interaction?

Don't let the distractions disrupt you from consistent physical activity. Remember that research shows that exercise can help you boost your mood, help you sleep better, help you keep a healthy weight, improve your immune system, digestive function, and your brain health, in addition to its impact the length of your telomere which can help you to slow down on aging and help you live a longer life.

Fill out Tables 1A and 1B and write down the number of distractions you had per day based on how you answered the questions on possible distractions or your own experience. When you track what you are doing, you put yourself in a better position to form the holistic habits that will help you improve.

Remind yourself of why you are doing this 30-day compass longevity challenge. You want to stay healthy so that so spend quality time with yourself, your family and your friends as you get older.

Is your mood one of the distractions that could be preventing you from having more consistent physical activity?

How can you walk more consistently? You can do this by setting daily objectives and the actions you can take to achieve those objectives. You can begin by finding simple but consistent ways to walk for about 30 minutes every day. If you don't have 30 minutes in one block, break up your exercise into 10 or 15 minutes each. Remember that 10 minutes of walking is about 1,000 steps. Since on average people have 2 to 2.5 feet per step, it takes about 2,000 steps to cover a mile. This means that 10,000 steps a day is about 5 miles a day

*Did you know that if you keep on putting off when you will exercise, you may end up not doing it?

My father in-law used to say that "Procrastination is the thief of time".

Don't procrastinate, do your exercise first in the morning or simply get up and do your exercise once the thought crosses your mind.

When you fill tables 1A and 1 B below, note how many days you failed to walk 10,000 steps , and how many distractions you had that day.

If you have not yet completed your 72-hour health and wellness complete audit by the 3rd of your 30-day longevity challenge.

TABLE 1A

Day	Number Of Steps	Minutes of walking	Jump Rope skips	Number of Push ups	Number of distractions
1					
2					
3					
4					
5					
6					
7					
8					
9					
10					
11					
12					
13					
14					
15					

.TABLE 1B

Day	Number Of Steps	Minutes of walking	Jump Rope skips	Number of Push ups	Number of distractions
16					
17					
18					
19					
20					
21					
22					
23					
24					
25					
26					
27					
28					
29					
30					

Day 3: Set the goal of losing one to two pounds every one to two weeks by walking

Specificity leads to focus. Remember that you need to set simple goals that you have the means to accomplish. This is part of the operational capacity of the compass profile. This is why on day 3 of your 30-day longevity challenge, I want you to set the specific goal of losing one and a quarter pounds per week through walking. Remember that maintaining a healthy weight is one keys to longevity.

How can you do this?

First weigh your yourself .

Second write the number of steps you take every day so that you will know what adjustments you need to make to help you lose one to two pounds every two weeks.

You can decide to try to lose weight by increasing your physical activity without making changes to your eating habits and improving your management of your stress-related and emotional challenges. How many steps a day do you need to lose 2.5 pounds in 2 weeks or 1.25 pounds in a week? Walking 1,000 steps a day would burn off about 50 calories, and 5000 steps would burn off about 250 calories per day, 35000 steps would only burn off 1750 calories a week and lead to losing 0.5 or half a pound a week.

If you want to lose 5 pounds in one month, it means you want to lose 2.5 pounds in 2 weeks, leading to 5 pounds in 4 weeks. You can lose 5 pounds in a month without changing much about what you eat by simply increasing the number of steps you take every day. If you used to walk only 5,000 steps a day, can you lose 2.5 pounds in a week? The answer would be No, because 5,000 steps a day would lead to losing 250 calories per day.

Research shows that 3,500 calories of energy equal 1 pound, but we need about 2,000 to 2,500 calories of energy for our usual daily activities. Therefore, you would have to starve or fast all day, in addition to exercising to have the energy deficit of 3,500 calories per day that will allow you to lose one pound a day. This is potentially dangerous, and it is usually not recommended or sustainable.

A less drastic and more sustainable approach would be to walk 10,000 steps per day so that you can burn off or lose 500 calories per day, leading to burning off about 3,500 calories per week or losing one pound per week by walking 70,000 steps per week.

While you can possibly lose one pound per week by walking 10,000 steps per day, if you find that your schedule makes this difficult, don't be discouraged. You can begin with doing 5,000 steps per day, which would lead to 35,000 steps per week or 70,000 steps in 2 weeks or burning off 3,500 calories in 2 weeks or losing one pound in 2 weeks.

Don't try to do all these calculations, just use a pedometer to track how many steps you are taking every day or every week. To lose one to two pounds in one to two weeks, you need to consistently walk 5,000 to 10,000 steps a day so that burn off about 250 calories to 500 calories per day. This is a simple sustainable way of losing about one to 2 pounds in 1 to 2 weeks.

Do you think you can walk 10,000 steps per day? If takes about 10 minutes to walk 1,000 steps, it means it will take about 100 minutes a day to walk 10,000 steps a day. Can you, do it? You can break your walks per day into 30 minutes or 10 to 15 minutes walk. A more realistic way of meeting your goal of regular physical activity for you might be to begin by finding simple but consistent ways to walk for about 30 minutes every day. If you don't have 30 minutes in one block, break up your exercise into 10 or 15 minutes each. Remember that 10 minutes of walking is about 1,000 steps. Since on average people have 2 to 2.5 feet per step, it takes about 2,000 steps to cover a mile. This means that 10,000 steps a day is about 5 miles a day.

The good news is that you can combine the steps from your formal physical activity period with the steps you take during activities like doing your chores, walking from one meeting to another, gardening or during other outdoor activities, to find out the total number of minutes, steps or miles, you have done in a day.

In this 30-day compass longevity challenge, continue to add at least 500 more steps per day, until you get to an average of 10,000 steps per day. If you are not getting to 10,000 steps per day, look at daily comments to see the adjustments you need to make.

Day 4: Use walking to meet a realistic goal of at least 50 minutes of daily physical activity

The task for day 4 of this 30-day compass longevity is meeting a goal of doing at least 50 minutes of physical activity every day through walking. Do you now consistently walk at least 10,000 steps a day? If you are walking at least 10,000 steps per day, then you are doing about 100 minutes of physical activity per day. Is this a realistic goal for you or do want to set a goal of about 5,000 steps a day to begin with? Even if you are able to walk only 5,000 steps, you are doing at least 50 minutes of physical activity per day.

How many minutes of physical activity do you need every week?

Keep in mind that the minimum moderate intensity such as walking, that was recommended by the WHO and the CDC is about 150 minutes per week or at least 30 minutes per day for 5 days in a week.

How many minutes of physical activities did you do today? Most guidelines recommend about 150 minutes per week of moderate physical activity. What does doing 150 minutes of exercise per week mean?
It means you are doing about 30 minutes of exercise per day for at least 5 days a week.

If your main exercise is walking, it means you are taking about 3000 steps per day since 1000 steps is equal to about 10 minutes of physical activity. Why is increasing your daily physical activity(PA) such an important part of making yourself healthier and living longer as you get older?

Research also shows that a sedentary lifestyle is considered a significant risk factor for cardiovascular disease while consistently doing more physical activity could be considered a non-pharmacological intervention for improving cardiovascular fitness in healthy and diseased individuals.

Your goal at the end of your 30-day longevity challenge should be walking at least 10,000 steps per day. On day one, find out the steps you walked. You can measure your steps per day with a pedometer or with a smart watch and get your average for the first 7 days then challenge yourself to meet up your goal by adding to your average in the next 7 days.

How will your realistic goals motivate you? They are achievable goals that can encourage you to become more active.

Don't allow daily distractions to prevent you from meeting your daily physical activity goals. Always strive to live a positive and fulfilled life.

Make sure you track your progress by filling table 2. You can even challenge yourself to walk at least 200 minutes every day. Keep in mind your operational capacity and your ambition profile. Use the resources you have and your goals realistic and achievable, one step at a time.

At 10 minutes per 1000 steps, 200 minutes of walking is 20,000 steps per day. You don't have to do the 200 minutes or 20,000 steps in one setting. You can strive to become more consistent with 10,000 steps in the first two weeks , then 12,500 in the third week, 15000 steps in the fourth week, or by 30 days.

What would you do if you were not able to get to 15,000 steps per day at the end of the first 30-day challenge? Begin another 30 - day challenge specifically for walking and try to do 5,000 steps in the first week, then 10,000 steps in the 2nd and 3rd week, then 15,000 steps in 4th week of your second 30-day challenge. .

TABLE 2

Day	Number Of Steps	Minutes of walking	Day	Number Of Steps	Minutes Of walking
1			16		
2			17		
3			18		
4			19		
5			20		
6			21		
7			22		
8			23		
9			24		
10			25		
11			26		
12			27		
13			28		
14			29		
15			30		

Day 5: Sleep at least 7 hours a day

*How many hours of sleep did you have today? Was it 5 hours of sleep, 6 hours , 7 hours or 8 hours?

*Write down how many hours of sleep you had on day 5. You can also write it down in your health and wellness journal or in your device or simple notebook you are using for doing your own 30 days longevity challenge.

Do you know why the number of hours you sleep every day can affect how long and healthy you will live? According to the CDC, 1 out of 3 adults do not get enough sleep or about 7 hours of sleep every night (CDC, 2016). According to the American Academy of Sleep Medicine and the Sleep Research Society, adults aged 18 to 60, need about 7 hours of sleep every night for great health and well-being. Sleeping less than 7 hours every night predisposes one to more chronic conditions like heart disease, diabetes, stroke, mental stress or depression, and obesity. This is consistent with the research that shows that there is an association between chronic poor sleep quality and an increased risk for age-related disease, mental health deterioration, and dying early (Sabot, Lovegrove, and Stapleton, 2023).

Do you know why having poor sleep predisposes one to poor health?

Here is an important integrative link, you can you use for your own compass blueprint for living a longer and better life. Research shows that inadequate sleep is associated with cellular damage through negative effects on telomere length (Sabot, Lovegrove, and Stapleton, 2023). Research also shows that sleep helps restore the body's nervous, immune, muscular, and skeletal systems. This restorative process is crucial for cognitive functions, such as emotional regulation and memory, and overall health and well-being (Sabot, Lovegrove, and Stapleton, 2023). The other thing to remember is that poor sleep includes the number of hours you have slept, how long it takes you to fall sleep and whether you wake up feeling rested or not.

Remember that the more you increase the amount of physical exercise that you participate in during the day, the easier it will be for you to sleep well. This is one of the keyways to help you get a good sleep at night. The more active your body is during the day, the more likely you are to relax at night and fall asleep faster.

If you doubt this, watch your children. You will find out that they sleep the most when they have been most busy running around and actively playing all day. They get into bed and fall sound asleep.

With regular exercise you'll notice that your quality of sleep is improved and the transition between the cycles and phases of sleep will become smoother and more regular. By keeping up your physical activity during the day, you may find it easier to deal with the stress and worries of your life.

*Write down how many steps you walked today. Did you walk at least 12,000 steps today? How many hours of sleep did you have today? The goal is to have 7 or more hours of sleep every day. How many hours did you spend on your TV or device?

During this 30-day compass longevity challenge your goal is that you increase the number of steps you take every day, reduce the number of hours you spend on TV and devices, and cut down disruptions like arguing, eating late or working late. Please fill out tables 3A and 3B, so that you can learn more about your sleeping pattern and adjustments you need to sleep more and adjustments you can make.

TABLE 3A

Day	Number Of Steps	Hours on TV	Number of Distractions	Hours of Sleep
1				
2				
3				
4				
5				
6				
7				
8				
9				
10				
11				
12				
13				
14				
15				

TABLE 3B

Day	Number Of Steps	Hours on TV	Number of Distractions	Hours of Sleep
16				
17				
18				
19				
20				
21				
22				
23				
24				
25				
26				
27				
28				
29				
30				

Day 6: Pay attention to the factors that can affect how well you sleep

Challenge yourself to go to bed on time and pay attention to the factors that can affect how well you sleep. If you work or play late into the night and end up being drained and confused the rest of the day, then you are ignoring your body clock for sleep, and it can affect your health and productivity at work. Get more hours of sleep, so that you can restore your body clock.

Are you a morning person, afternoon person or night person? A friend of mine who was a night person had a hard time adjusting to waking up at 4.a.m., every morning to catch the 5 a.m. bus that would take him to Los Angeles for his morning shift, until he summoned the courage to ask his supervisor for a change to night shift.

Paying attention to these factors can help you make your life healthier. Why? This is because your body depends on an intricate circadian rhythm to function well. It needs adequate sleep, nutrition, and shelter to stay optimal. It also depends on your priorities and how you schedule your activities.

Do you go to bed with your phone or computer in your hand or on your bed?

Do you sleep once you lie in bed, or do you take time to sleep?

Write down what time you ate before you went to bed.

How many times do you dream when you sleep?

Do you travel a lot as part of your daily activity? How do you handle travel that may affect your body clock? You have to schedule adequate sleep and rest, so that you do not end up getting stressed out and putting in sub-optimal performance. It can affect your outcome and sense of fulfillment. One way to overcome this is to make relentless transformation your priority.

The more you understand the ways your body clock affects your health and energy level, the more you can share the knowledge with your spouse, friends, and family. This is part of the process of increasing your self-mastery and helping yourself live a longer and healthier life!

How many times did you wake up at night? Fill up tables 4A and 4B to get more details about your sleeping pattern and the adjustments you can make as part of your sleeping pattern. If you stay up late or play late into the night and end up being drained and confused the rest of the day, then you are ignoring your body clock for sleep, and it can affect your health and productivity at work. Get more hours of sleep, so that you can restore your body clock.

TABLE 4A

Day	How many times did you wake up at night? day	How many times did go to bed with device in your hand?	Number of Dreams	Hours of Sleep
1				
2				
3				
4				
5				
6				
7				
8				
9				
10				
11				
12				
13				
14				
15				

TABLE 4B

Day	How many times did you wake up at night? day	How many times did go to bed with device in your hand?	Number of Dreams	Hours of Sleep
16				
17				
18				
19				
20				
21				
22				
23				
24				
25				
26				
27				
28				
29				
30				

TABLE 4C

Day	Did you travel?	What time did you come back from work?	What time did you eat before sleeping?	Hours of Sleep
1				
2				
3				
4				
5				
6				
7				
8				
9				
10				
11				
12				
13				
14				
15				

TABLE 4D

Day	Did you travel?	What time did you come back from work?	What time did you eat before sleeping?	Hours of Sleep
16				
17				
18				
19				
20				
21				
22				
23				
24				
25				
26				
27				
28				
29				
30				

Day 7: Set realistic goals for achieving consistent 7 hours or more of sleep every day

From days 5 and 6 of this 30-day longevity challenge, you now know how many hours of sleep you have every day and the factors that affect how well you sleep. Now you have to make adjustments based on what you have found out and try to consistently sleep for 7 or more hours every day.

Write down how many hours of sleep you had on day 7. As we get older, we discover that sleep does not come as readily as in the past Remember that the more physical activity you have during the day, the more likely you will have hours of sleep every day.

Increase your number of steps per day by at least 20% per day till you start doing 10,000 steps per day consistently. This means that if you were doing an every of 5,000 steps per day in the last 7 days, your goal in the next 7 days will be 1,000 steps per day, till you get to 10,000 steps a day. .

Cut down on the hours or minutes you spend on your devices per day.

Don't eat late at night, especially if you notice that when you eat late at night , you end up having less than 7 hours of sleep.

Don't lie in bed with your phone. Set the goal of doing this for the next 7 days. If you do it write down why, and the changes you need to make.

Don't allow others to make you so mad or so worried that you spend your night lying in bed without sleeping. Set the goal of giving yourself positive self-talk that will help let go of your worries or manage your stressors and sleep. These are all distractions. The problem is that inadequate sleep will eventually affect your health and productivity, if you don't take consistent action.

Don't forget that in order to achieve your goals you must have daily objectives and targets that represent mini steps towards accomplishing your goals or projects, that you actually take or do.

*How many times were you distracted enough not to sleep at least 7 hours a day in the past 72 hours?

What is your 30-day sleep challenge? How many hours of sleep do you have every day? Is it 5 hours a day, 6 hours a day or at least 7 hours a day? Record your first 7 days, then the next 7 days, then try to maintain an average of 7 hours a day at the end of your 30-day challenge. What percentage of days do you sleep at least 7 hours? Is it at least up to 80% of days in your 30-day challenge? While 100% is preferred, 80% at least meets the 80:20 rule.

Day 8: Pay attention to your blood pressure and your numbers

Are you healthy or do you simply feel healthy without truly knowing if you are healthy or not? Do you know your blood pressure? **Do you know your numbers?** Knowing your numbers is part of the Compass metabolic and physical profiles.

Please write down your weight, height and BMI. If you don't know your numbers or have not had a physical this year, please see your doctor and have one. When was the last time you checked your blood pressure or went for a physical?

Even if you had previously weighed yourself or day 2, weigh yourself again on day 8.

Write down your weight and waist circumference. If you are feeling healthy but you don't know your blood pressure, how do you know that you are healthy.

Do you know if your blood pressure is 110/70mmHg or 130/80mmHg or 200/110mmHg? High blood pressure is one the most common chronic conditions that can affect your health and longevity?

The previous guidelines considered a blood pressure of 140/90 mmHg to be high blood pressure but since 2017 the new AHA guidelines defined high blood pressure as a reading of 130/80 mmHg and anything between 120 to 129 mm Hg as elevated.

If your blood pressure is 190/100mmHg and you didn't know it, you're a ticking time bomb for a major life altering or possibly life-ending event like a stroke or heart attack. A few years ago, a 53-year-old man, who was in apparent good health or felt healthy collapsed and died after a failed resuscitation. Before he died, EMT found out that his blood pressure was 260/150 mmHg , and he had had a heart attack while exercising. His wife, who was with him in the gym when he collapsed, said he had always been in relatively good health and was not on any medications.

This example of someone dying while exercising is important because too many people think that simply because they exercise regularly, eat healthy, sleep well and have no symptoms, then they must be in good health. If you ask them their blood pressure or weight, they won't know. They will tell you they don't need to do anything or worry because they are doing well and do not need to do anything else. This is a wrong and potentially deadly assumption. High blood pressure is a silent killer, you could have it without having symptoms.

You need to know your own numbers. You need to have an idea of the potential illnesses you could be dealing with as you get older based on your family history, past medical history and age group. Do you know your family history? Do you have diabetes, high blood pressure or kidney disease in your family? Do you know the commonest cause of illness or death in your age group as you get older? If you want to live longer, it is important that you pay attention to what has happened to others or is happening to most people your age.

For this challenge, all you need to do is to measure your blood pressure every day for the next 30 days and make comments about whether you did or did not. Fill Table 5.In the comments write down if you slept well or not, write down how many hours you slept, what was your compass stress index for the day, and did you eat five servings of fruits and vegetables? If you have not yet done your yearly physical or gone for your yearly check up with your primary care provider, do it.

TABLE 5

Day	Blood Pressure	Day	Blood Pressure	Comments
1		16		
2		17		
3		18		
4		19		
5		20		
6		21		
7		22		
8		23		
9		24		
10		25		
11		26		
12		27		
13		28		
14		29		
15		30		

Day 9: Make sure you are managing the leading causes of death for your age group

What are the leading causes of death for those 50 and above? **Worldwide leading causes of death for older people are the following:**

Heart disease
Stroke
COPD
Lower respiratory infections.

You need to pay attention to the common causes of death and illness for your age group. According to the National Council on Aging (NCOA) the leading causes of death among older people in the US are heart disease, cancer, C0VID-19, stroke, chronic lower respiratory diseases, Alzheimer's, and diabetes (NCOA,2023).

US leading causes of death for older people are the following:

Heart disease
Cancer
COVID-19
Stroke
Chronic lower respiratory diseases
Alzheimer's
Diabetes

The interesting thing about this is that 5 years ago or in 2018, it would not have included COVID 19. This shows one of the reasons why everyone must remain vigilant. Things change, and we have to learn to take notice and make our own adjustments.

According to the WHO, the leading causes of death among older people, worldwide are **heart disease, stroke, chronic obstructive pulmonary disease, and lower respiratory infections (WHO, 2020).** We need to keep these leading causes of death or illness in mind when making our own health and wellness decisions and actions.

How can you make sure you are managing the leading causes of death for your age group? Go and see your doctor and get your labs done. Write your blood pressure and weight. Make a note of what part of your family history or even your medical history you need to pay particular attention to.

*Write down your blood sugar or find out your blood sugar level.
*Do you smoke? You need to stop smoking.
*How many cigarettes did you smoke today?
*How much alcohol did you drink today?

If you have not yet done a medical or health checkup or physical in years and you have no idea what your blood pressure is or what your weight, blood sugar or cholesterol level, then your physical.

Have you done your age-related screening tests like your PSA or colonoscopy?

How many medications did you take today? Write down how many medications you took today.

Are you struggling with remembering things?

Please, don't make the mistake of assuming that because you are not on any medications, and you don't have any symptoms of illness, and you haven't been to the doctor in years and are feeling well, then you must be healthy. This is not always true. If you don't have concrete data and verified medical opinion telling you that your health status is good, don't assume you have optimal health.

How many times have you heard about someone who was healthy and working out regularly and was full of life, who suddenly slumped and died? How many times did the news report also state that the person had high blood pressure but didn't know? One way to help yourself minimize the risk of such an experience is to begin your own journey towards using integrative strategies , and simple habits and ways to have a more consistent healthy lifestyle.

Go and see your doctor and get some labs done to get a data-based health assessment of your health status. Do you know your blood sugar level? Do you know your cholesterol level? How well are your kidneys and liver functioning?

Let's face it! Most of us think we are very healthy. This is a common thought for young adults and those in their middle age. Yet we all know that looks can be deceiving. I am sure you have all heard stories of people who were apparently very healthy then suddenly died from a heart attack or cancer after a "brief illness" or even had a near death experience (NDE).

The most important task on day 9 is for you to see your doctor and follow up on the common causes of death for your age group and get your blood work done. During your 30-day longevity challenge make sure you are paying daily attention to the common causes of death for your age group.

Day 10: Natural ways you can improve your heart health

What is the challenge for day 10 of the 30-day longevity challenge? The challenge is paying more attention to your heart health. Go for your regular check-up with your doctor or healthcare provider and make changes to your lifestyle that can help you improve your heart health. Do you know that there are natural ways you can improve your heart health?

What do you need to know? You need to know that heart disease is among the leading causes of death for middle-aged men and women in most parts of the world, including the United States and Western Europe. Even in developing countries like Nigeria the trend toward more deaths related to heart disease is becoming more common.

Have you measured your blood pressure in the past 7 days? As part of this 30-day compass longevity challenge you should have measured your blood pressure by day 3. If you haven't, measure it today and measure it every other day or as directed by your doctor. Start your own blood pressure log or review the 72-hour health and wellness audit that you did before.

Do you know the factors that could affect your blood pressure and heart health?

Poorly managed stress
Daily anger
Making unhealthy food choices
Poor self-care-Not taking your medications, after a diagnosis of high blood pressure or diabetes
Poor weight management-not maintaining a healthy weight
Family history of high blood pressure

Do you have any friends that suddenly had a stroke or died from heart attack?

Do you have any friends, relatives, colleagues, or siblings that unexpectedly had heart attacks and survived? This what I typically call a near death experience (NDE).

Do you want to have your own NDE, before you begin to take the steps that will help you to reduce your cardiovascular risk factors and improve your own heart health?

You can improve your heart health by finding natural ways to reduce your cardiovascular risk factors.

*Do you know the factors that can affect your heart health?

The factors include the following:

Age
Sex
Weight
Blood pressure
Blood sugar
Smoking
Drinking alcohol

Family History
Triglyceride Level
HDL or good cholesterol
LDL or bad cholesterol

High blood pressure, stroke and heart attack and other related heart diseases are common problems that you could experience as you get older. What are you going to do about them?

*Do you know your blood pressure today?

Some natural ways you can reduce your blood pressure or keep it at about 120/80 mmHg, will be to first measure it, watch what you eat, cut down on your sodium intake, manage stress better, exercise more, and live more of a telomeric lifestyle.

*Weigh yourself and write down your weight today. This is an example of how knowing your numbers can affect different aspects of your health.

Would you not like to know what is your probability or chances of having a heart attack in the next 10 years?

*Do you know how much sodium you eat daily? If you don't know, read your nutrition facts to get an idea of how much sodium you eat every day, then reduce it.

The problem is that most of us still feel that heart attacks and NDEs are things that happen to others. We do not feel it will happen to us, so we take little or no precautions to modify our risks for such adverse health events.

You can reduce your risk of having heart disease and other related NDEs by reducing your LDL level and increasing your HDL. Getting more details about your lipid-profile and other blood work is part of the compass metabolic profile, which is the fifth component of the compass profiles.

*Write down the last time you saw your doctor or did your blood work? Do you know your lipid profile? Do you know your cholesterol level? If you don't know your cholesterol and you are 40 and above you are making a big mistake, because some health associations recommend that people should start doing a check of their cholesterol level from 20 years of age. Knowing your lipid profile is important because you can use it in computing your cardiovascular risk. Your lipid profile includes your triglyceride level, total cholesterol, HDL (High Density Lipoprotein) or good cholesterol, and LDL (Low density Lipoprotein) or bad cholesterol.

Do you know changes you can make to eating and healthy living habits that will help you reduce your bad cholesterol (LDL) and increase your good cholesterol(HDL)?
Here are some ways you can help yourself reduce your LDL or bad cholesterol. First, you can add chia seeds to your daily meal. The great thing about chia seeds is that you can add them to almost anything you eat. You can add them to your oatmeal, brown rice, salad, or yoghurt. **Chia seeds contain a lot of soluble fibers that can help you**

lower your cholesterol. Eat more fiber! How much fiber do you eat daily? Unless you switch to fiber-rich carbohydrate sources like baked sweet potato, whole grain bread, barley, oatmeal, and brown rice, you may end up quitting after a few weeks.

Generally speaking, our focus is on fiber content of the food rather than on glycemic index. That is why the challenge for day 18 of the 30-day compass longevity challenge is eating at least 50g of fiber every day.

Here is a simple way you can easily eat 50g of fiber every day. Eat more fiber by more chia seeds every day. Chia seeds contain a lot of fiber, and you should them part of the variety in your healthy eating. Eat more fruits, vegetables, and fibers as fillers. Fibers are especially good for your system because they help to increase bowel movement. This has the added effect of making your digestive system more efficient.

*Write down how many eggs you ate today.

*** How many eggs did you eat in the past 7 days?** If you don't know, go and check your health wellness journal or do a 72- hour food audit to find out.

The second thing you can do is to cut down on the number of eggs you eat if you are eating too many eggs a day. Though eggs are low in carbs, rich in protein and lutein, eggs also have about 180 mg of cholesterol depending on the size of egg. Eating more egg white, instead of egg yolk will help you cut down on dietary cholesterol.

How many eggs a day is healthy? Current research suggests that eating an egg a day or about 7 eggs per week is healthy for most people. According to Harvard Health, research now shows that the amount of cholesterol you eat does not directly affect the cholesterol in your body, because most of the cholesterol in your body is made the liver and it is the saturated fat in your diet that can make your live make more cholesterol. According to the Heart Foundation New Zealand, the saturated fatty acids in our diets has a greater effect on blood levels of cholesterol and possibly related heart disease.

Today is the 10th day of your 30-day longevity challenge. What are the average number of steps you have taken in the past 9 or 10 days? The third thing you can do is to increase your daily physical activity to at least 50 minutes per day. Increase in daily physical activity improves quality of life, reduces body weight, reduces LDL cholesterol, increases HDL cholesterol, increases insulin sensitivity, and helps to prevent pathologic conditions like obesity, atherosclerosis, diabetes, and decreases blood pressure both at rest and during exercise, thus helping to prevent metabolic syndrome and a hypertensive state (Sorriento, Vaia and Iaccarino, 2021)

What are the benefits of reducing your LDL or bad cholesterol level? According to the CDC, too much LDL can build up in our blood vessels and lead to the buildup of plaque which can increase the risk of heart disease and stroke. This means that high levels of LDL can affect your vascular health. One of the benefits of cutting down LDL is the reduced risk that follows.

In this compass longevity challenge, the focus will be on asking yourself if you are regularly doing the things that will help to lower your LDL, reduce your total triglycerides and increase your HDL.

What is your main task for the 10th of the 30-day compass longevity of challenge? Challenge yourself to consistently do the physical activity that will help lower bad cholesterol and increase good cholesterol, while increasing your daily fiber intake to about 50g per day. Make sure that you regularly do your labs and lipide profile through your doctor.

TABLE 6A

Day	Number Of Steps	Average daily grams of fiber	Number of servings of fruits and Veggies	Compass Stress Index (CSI)
1				
2				
3				
4				
5				
6				
7				
8				
9				
10				
11				
12				
13				
14				
15				

TABLE 6B

Day	Number Of Steps	Average daily grams of fiber	Number of servings of fruits and Veggies	Compass Stress Index (CSI)
16				
17				
18				
19				
20				
21				
22				
23				
24				
25				
26				
27				
28				
29				
30				

Day 11: Calculate your own cardiovascular risk factor

On day 11 of the 30 -day compass longevity challenge you will learn how calculate your own cardiovascular risk factor. The factors that you can use to calculate your cardiovascular risk factor include the following:
 *Age
*Sex
*Race
 *Family history of heart disease or diabetes
*Lipid profile as stated above.
 *BMI
*Personality type
Age, sex, and race are factors that cannot usually be changed, but you can use them to calculate your cardiovascular risk points and then convert the points to percentage risk for heart attack over a 10-year period.

Here is an example of the cardiovascular points for a 45- year-old- man Benjamin with a low HDL(<35) and a cholesterol of 220 and a blood pressure of 130/80 mmHg, who is not diabetic but smokes. Being a 45-year-old male, would give him 6 points, if he was a woman the points would be 5. An HDL of less than 35 would give him 2 points. Total cholesterol of 220 would be equivalent to 2 points. Smoking would give him 4 points, while a blood pressure of 130/80mmHg is equivalent to 3 points.

This calculation means Joseph has (6+2+2+4+3)=17 points and would translate to at least 29.4% risk of cardiovascular disease(CVD) in 10 years .What does this mean?

According to the Framingham Heart Study, moderate risk is a 10-year CVD risk of less than 10%, moderately high risk is 10-20% and high risk is 20%and above. This means that Benjamin has a high risk for cardiovascular disease. For Benjamin the man in this example, his numbers mean that 29 out of 100 people with his risk profile

will have a heart attack in the next 10 years
This is too high a risk as confirmed by the
Framingham Heart Study.

The advantage of finding out your risk
factor before having a heart attack is that it
gives you an opportunity to take action.
What is the benefit of having high HDL?

According to the CDC , HDL or high
density lipoprotein helps to move
cholesterol from the blood to the liver. This
means a higher level of HDL would help to
reduce the risk of heart disease and stroke.
For Benjamin he can change his risk for a
heart disease by quitting smoking, this will
take away,4 points from his 17. Making his
HDL 50 and his total cholesterol less than
160, would give him points of (-1), and (0).
This means his new total CVD points will be
(6+(-1)+0+0+3)=8, which will be equivalent
to 6.7%,10-year risk of CVD. Essentially
this means that by taking action and
modifying his risk factors through eating
healthier and quitting smoking, Benjamin
reduced his risk of having a heart attack by
more than half.

He changed his risk of a heart attack from 29 out of 100 people in 10 years to 7 out of 100 people in 10 years, for people with a similar heart risk profile. Wow! I hope you are as excited as I am; with just a few changes to our eating habits and lifestyle changes we can minimize our risk for a life-threatening event like a heart attack. Do these numbers and percentages look confusing or interesting?

Do not worry, it is not that confusing. You can calculate your own personal risk of having a heart attack by visiting http://hp2010.nhlbihin.net/atpiii/calculator.asp or simply using the following calculator: Framingham Risk Calculator (omnicalculator.com)

2018 Prevention Guidelines Tool CV Risk Calculator (heart.org)

The 30-day longevity challenge is for you to start working on lowering your cardiovascular risk factor after the initial calculation on day 11.

Day 12: 5 simple steps you need to challenge yourself to take every day to help you manage the chronic conditions that could shorten your life

Day 12 is the day you challenge yourself to begin to take the 5 simple steps every day that will help to manage the chronic conditions that could shorten your life. The first simple step you need to take every day is to lower the expectations that you have when you are interacting with others.

Be careful not to expect too much from others, so that you won't be disappointed, or become resentful or angry when their behavior is different from what you expect. Research has shown that lowering expectations can reduce disappointment and increase health and happiness. Your own daily happiness will depend on if things are going better than expected or worse than expected. When things are going worse than expected you will be sad and angry and end up with too many negative emotions which will not be good for your health. When things go better than expected you will have more positive emotions and less chronic inflammation which will be great for your health.

When you start your day with lower expectations in terms of what others would do, or how they would react to what you say or act, you will be less disappointed or stressed out during your interactions with them. How many times did you lower expectations during your interactions with others today? Do you always lower your expectations during your interactions with others so that you do not get so stressed out and disappointed by what others are doing that you no longer enjoy the moment?

The second simple step is focusing on what you can control. Don't waste your time and your energy on what you cannot control. You cannot control what people will say or do, but you can control how you will use your time or how you will react. Don't get yourself worked up because the person you are talking to is not listening to you.

The third simple step is walking 10,000 steps a day. This is part of making sure you do at least 50 minutes of exercise every day. Decide to apply the 80:20 rule to your exercise regimen. This means you have to decide and follow through on doing consistent physical activity. Don't try to do everything. Find 1 out of 5 and do it 80% of the time. Walking is strongly recommended.

The fourth simple step is eating healthy every day. Remember healthy eating is one of the ways you can improve your heart health. Don't try to eat all veggies and fruits, find about 3 of 15 that you eat 80 % of the time. You can begin by eating more fruits and vegetables like apples, cucumbers and colorful vegetables. Eat every meal with veggies, fruits and fiber.

Make sure you actually eat something you actually like. If you don't settle on a fruit or vegetable that you enjoy eating after a while you will give up. **One of the aims of this 30-day challenge is to help you form sustainable holistic habits that will help you live a longer and better life.**

The fifth simple step is to become better at positively managing the patterns that dominate your daily life so that you can become a better version of yourself every day. This is tantamount to seeking continuous self-improvement and maintaining a positive outlook no matter what. Don't let the situation or what others say get to you or rob you of your confidence

What are the patterns you commonly encounter in your daily life? Write down the patterns that are most prominent in your life in the past 72 hours or 7 days. You can write this down in your "Guide to Aging Well" journal or Wellness journal. Identify and write down the following with regards to you:

*Eating pattern
*Working pattern
*Communication pattern

*Decision making pattern
***Relationship pattern**
Are your relationships positive and supportive?
*** Stress pattern**
What is the biggest source of stress for you? Is it conversational or not?
***Conflict pattern**
Are you easily irritated or angry?
Do you always have to be right? Are all others fools simply because they are not as successful as yourself?
***Self-mastery pattern**
What purpose drives your actions? Are your actions driven by your relationship to a higher power, the universe, God, humanity or simply your desire for excellence and self-preservation ? Know yourself.

Why are patterns important? Through them you will get a better idea of the habits that are driving your daily action and lifestyle, and the changes you need to make to increase your self-accountability and self-mastery.

Do you have a pattern of postponing seeing your doctor and taking your medications? Do your lab tests if you haven't done them. Keep your doctor's appointment. Take your medications. Finally make sure you also apply the 80:20 rule to managing stress, maintaining your own positive and supportive relationships and improving your self-care. Remember that to foresee is to rule.

What is your 30-day longevity managing chronic conditions challenge? First write down the chronic conditions that you know of in the first 7 days. If you don't know any, start by checking your blood pressure and weighing yourself weekly. The second step is to go to your doctor and find out if you have any chronic conditions that you may not be aware of. At the end of the 30-day challenge, you will know how many of the steps recommended in this chapter have been consistently taking and which ones you need to continue to improve on. After all as the great Dala Omeokachie said, "Improvement never ends."

Day 13: Make more healthy food choices by cutting down on processed food and eating more plant-based food

Do you know that you can live a healthier longer life by cutting down on processed food and eating more plant-based food ?

*Have you done your 72- hour food audit to get an idea of the food choices you typically make?

*What did you eat last night?

*Do you eat a lot of processed food? Keep in mind that not all processed food is bad after all by definition any food that has been deliberately altered before we eat is processed food.

Cut down or completely stop eating processed meats like bacon, hot dogs, sausage, and ham. Do you know that eating processed meats has been associated with a higher risk of getting colorectal cancer? Yet when you go to outdoor events, hot dogs with all sorts of dressings are among the most commonly severed meals.

If you don't keep your eye and your mind on what you eat, no one else will do it for you. The sad thing is that if you get ill from eating food that you could have avoided eating, all those friends that were hanging out with you when you were having a good time won't be with you in that hospital bed, when you will be dealing with illnesses that unhealthy food choices could have contributed to.

If you haven't done your 72 – hour food audit, do it or go back to your health and wellness journal to find out your eating pattern and food choices. This will help you decide the changes you need to make to help you eat healthy and make the healthy food choices that will help you live a healthier and longer life

Why would making healthy food choices and eating less processed food and more fruits and vegetables help you to live longer? According to the Global Burden of Disease study, 1 in 5 deaths in the world can be prevented by eating healthy or improving the quality of diet. One way to simply do this is to eat more plant-based food and cut down on processed food.

The other problem with eating processed food is that generally speaking, the more processed food you eat, the higher the glycemic index of the food you are eating. While it is good to know about different ways, what we eat can impact our health, sometimes when you find a way to eat healthy that verifiably works for you without the knowledge of all other terms and ways of classifying healthy food. What may matter more is your consistency in eating right. Fast when you can or when it is safe for you do so and make more of your food more plant-based, while watching your portions and snacks.

If you want to live longer one of the healthy food choices you can make is to cut down on drinking sugary drinks or sugar-sweetened beverages like soda, fruit juice, and fruit punch. According to CDC sugar-sweetened beverages (SSBs) or sugary drinks like sodas are leading sources of added sugars in the American diet. Drinking soda is associated with weight gain/obesity, type 2 diabetes, gout, tooth decay, heart disease, kidney diseases, and liver disease (CDC, 2017). **Drink water or unsweetened tea instead of soda.**

How many times do you drink fruit juice in a day?

How many times do you drink soda in a day?

One of the ways you can make sure that you eat more plant-based food is to eat more fruits and vegetables. Do you eat cucumbers, cabbages, green leaf, tomatoes, broccoli, oranges, mangoes, apples, pineapples, grapes, and blueberries? If these do not work for you, make your own list. Make changes for the ones you don't like. Some people prefer carrots to mangoes. Make your own list and regularly eat them or regularly make fruit and vegetable smoothies from them. You can try the blueberry and cucumber smoothie made with grapes and bananas. It is delicious and smooth!

You need to remember that eating healthy through cutting down on processed food and eating more plant-based food will you help maintain a healthy weight, which can help you to reduce the effect of being overweight or obese on your lifespan. Research shows that having excessive weight can lead to increase in insulin resistance, inflammation, and metabolic and hormonal changes that can lead to neurodegeneration, atherosclerosis and a tendency to produce tumors.

Research also shows that increasing body mass index (BMI) increases the risk of developing type 2 diabetes, cancer and cardiovascular disease. In addition to being associated with the above listed changes, having excessive fat which is both a function of how you eat and how consistently you exercise can increase the risk of having coronary disease, high blood pressure, nonalcoholic liver disease, stroke , type 2 diabetes and aging at a faster rate.

Have you done your 72- hour food audit to get an idea of the food choices you typically make? What did you eat last night? Do you eat a lot of processed food? If you haven't done your 72 – hour food audit, do it or go back to your health and wellness journal to find out your eating pattern and food choices. This will help you decide the changes you need to make to help you eat healthy and make the food choices that will help you live a healthier and longer life.

Your goal should be to make healthy food choices at least 80% of the time, in the next 30 days, starting from today.

Day 14: Eating in moderation and intermittent fasting

On day 14 of the 30-day compass longevity challenge, your focus should be on eating in moderation. While there are many ways to eat in moderation, I will share with you how to use the compass intermittent fasting healthy eating plan and the compass VAM method to eat in moderation.

Please don't do intermittent fasting without first talking to your doctor or provider. Don't do intermittent fasting if you are trying to conceive, pregnant or nursing. Intermittent fasting is broadly defined as any diet or eating plan that includes regular periods of not eating or fasting.

In this 30-day compass longevity challenge, I will show you how to use the 16:8 type of intermittent fasting. In this type you fast for

16 hours then you eat in 8 hours. When you are following the 16:8 intermittent fasting type, you will fast for 16 hours a day, and have the remaining 8 hours to eat. With intermittent fasting you can easily cut down your caloric intake without counting calories. Intermittent fasting has also been found to be one of the healthy, safe and easy ways to lose 1-2 lbs. per week without counting calories.

Research shows that intermittent fasting works by extending the time the body has burned through the calories consumed in your last meal and begins to burn fat in lieu of consumed calories (John Hopkins, 2022). You have to remember that the period of fasting could lead to even more hunger pangs, tiredness, loss of concentration, and weakness. The good news is that during the fasting period, you can drink water, black coffee, and unsweetened tea. Personally, I start my day with black coffee, it helps to keep me sharp and alert as I go through my day.

Do you drink coffee in the morning? You will require some discipline to make sure that you manage the hunger pangs during the fasting period well. Don't eat too much during the eating phase of intermittent fasting.

If you are doing a 16-8 hour, intermittent fasting, you take your last meal on or before 8pm, and eat your breakfast at noon the following day or eat last meal or snacks for the day at 10 pm, then first meal of the next day at 2pm or later.

*Watch the portion of the food you eat.

*Watch the type of food you eat.

***Don't drink soda or eat hot dogs as an immediate way of dealing with your hunger pangs.**

Remember that research has shown that eating healthy is one of the ways you can potentially reduce the shortening of the length of telomeres in your cells, leading to delayed onset of age-related diseases and increased longevity or lifespan (Shamas,2011).You can make changes to your eating habits through the compass vam method.

VAM, in the compass vam method stands for variety, adjustments, and moderation. Begin eating in moderation by reducing the food portion of your daily meals.

***Cut down the servings or portions of your regular meal by half.** This will reduce your energy intake by about half or a third. You fill the gap with vegetables and fruits. If you feel pangs of hunger, snack with nuts, drink plenty of water or eat some fruits.

Why is the reduction in portions so important? According to surveys by doctors and nutritionists the average American male takes about 3,000 calories per day and the American female about 2,400 calories per day (Reuters Health, 2015). According to Dr. Wang an energy intake and expenditure expert, consistent loss, or reduction in energy intake of 100 calories would lead to

---

10 pounds loss in weight in about year (Reuters Health, 2015).

The more you reduce your servings, the more weight you would lose because the fewer calories you will take in, the less excess calories you will have to store as fat.

Do you check the calories in your food? **You do not have to do a full detailed calories count to know your average energy intake. You can get a good idea of your calories intake by doing your own 72-hour food audit. This will help you identify the highest and most frequent source of calories in your daily meals.**

All you have to do is to remember that you have to reduce all sources of your daily intake of calories from your meals to your snacks. Do this to a level that allows you to feel full, eat healthy and still lose weight. Remember that it is calories in, calories out!

Make sure the food you eat every day contains adequate but moderate portions

of fat, proteins, carbohydrates and vitamins. Eat enough food to fill full when you eat. If you don't feel full after a meal you will find yourself eating too many sugary snacks in between meals to make you feel full. One trick is to drink a glass of water before every meal, it will help you to feel full with every meal.

Make sure you drink at least one glass of water before and after a meal. This is important because eating only up to 80 % full was one of the common practices of people of Okinawa in Japan, who have the highest number of centenarians in the world (Boyle & Long, 2010).

Okinawa is one of the so-called blue zones in the world where a lot of people live up to 100 years or more. If you want to lose weight or manage your weight better without making it seem like a tedious task, then drink at least two glasses of water per meal and increase the bulk in your meals through fruits and vegetables. **This will help you reduce your total calorie intake per**

meal without torture diets or counting calories

If you are eating in moderation by cutting down your portions, eating fruits and vegetables and doing regular exercise but have not lost weight, you wonder why. It could be that you have cut down on your portions, increased your food variety and may have started over snacking.

Be careful with snacks!!!Pay careful attention to size or frequency of your snacks, because you may still be eating a lot of calories per day through snacks

The main task of day 14 of the compass longevity challenge is combining intermittent fasting with reducing the portion of food you eat per meal. Before you start intermittent fasting ask your doctor. If you can't do intermittent fasting, use the above strategies to continue to eat in moderation. Starting today, and in the next 30 days, you need to make sure you follow through with the eat in moderation strategies discussed above.

Day 15: Make sure you use your nutrition facts every day

One of the important adjustments you can make to your healthy eating is to read your nutrition facts so that you can know what you are eating per serving size, and what adjustments you need to make.

On Day 15 of your 30-day longevity challenge, make sure you are reading the nutritional facts on the food that you are eating. This will help you make sure that you are eating the right portion of the food that you want to it and that you know how much sodium, potassium and added sugar you are getting in the food you are eating.

Did you check the nutritional facts in the food you are eating today? Make sure you make reading your nutritional facts one of your daily habits .

Through reading the Nutrition Fact label on your food , you will be able to find out the following:

Calories per serving size
Added sugar per serving size
Fiber per serving size
Sodium per serving size
Potassium per serving size
Saturated Fat per serving size
Protein per serving size

When you regularly read the nutrition facts in the food you eat, you can find out calories per serving. When you know the calories per serving you can more realistically adjust your portion size to cut down on your daily calories intake without counting calories

Make sure before you eat that you check the Nutrition Facts in every food that you eat. Make sure you always check for added sugar in what you eat.

According to the CDC sugar-sweetened beverages (SSBs) or sugary drinks like sodas are leading sources of added sugars in the American diet. Drinking soda is associated with weight gain/obesity, type 2 diabetes, gout, tooth decay, heart disease, kidney diseases, and liver disease (CDC, 2017).

If you want to live longer of the healthy food choices you can make to drinking sugary drinks or sugar-sweetened beverages like soda, fruit-juice, and fruit punch. **Drink water or unsweetened tea instead of soda**

Write down many cans of energy drink do you drink every day.

How many cups of water do you drink every day?
How many slices of bread do you eat every day?
Do you eat 4 slices of bread a day or more?

Do you eat 8 slices of bread a day?

Did you know that bread can be a source of sodium and too much energy intake?

Did you know that on average a slide of bread contains 150 mg of sodium and 110 calories per serving? This would mean that for bread with one slice per serving, 10 slices would be 1100calories. This would be more than half of the average 2000 calories per day recommended for most people.

The second reason may be related to your snacking habits. Did you know that one small pack of unsalted pea nuts contained 220 calories per serving but 6 servings per pack? How does this information which you read from the nutrition facts on the pack help you? It can help you determine calories per pack, sodium per pack and sugar per pack.

If you are eating a lot of nuts, check your nutritional facts as soon as possible. Don't assume that one bag of nuts is the serving size. You could have a bag of nuts with 3 serving sizes. This means that if the bag has 90 mg of sodium per serving size, then you eat the whole bag of nuts in one sitting, you have actually eaten (3X90)mg or 270 mg of sodium instead of 90 mg of sodium. If you have high blood pressure or even pre-hypertensive, not paying close attention to your nutrition facts could lead to an accounted source of more sodium than you would have preferred in your daily meal.

When was the last time you checked your nutritional facts before you ate your meal? Form the new habit of checking your nutritional facts by adding it to one the things you will track through your habit tracker.

Do you check the fat in the milk you drink? Do you drink whole mile, 2% reduced milk , or fat free milk?

You can also gradually reduce the fat content in your milk products. You can do this by changing the variety of milk that you drink from whole milk to 2% fat: then to 1% fat. I am wary of fat free milk because it is still important to get fat in your body which can be used through cellular metabolism to produce cell membranes and hormones. More specifically cholesterol is used through cellular metabolism to produce cell membranes and hormones.

Aim to reduce your fat intake rather than avoiding fat altogether. Eat lower-fat cheese and yogurt. When you buy yogurt, also check that it does not contain sugar. The good thing about changing to 1% fat milk is that it remains tasty. Fat has 9 calories of energy per gram compared to carbohydrates and proteins that have about 4 per gram. This makes fat one of the more efficient ways your body can store energy. This is one of the reasons why excess calories end up being stored as fat your body. Through regular reading of nutritional facts you pay closer attention to carbs per serving and sugar per serving.

Remember calories in calories out. However, it is better when those calories contain fibers too. An easy way to add fiber to your meal is to add Chia seeds to your meal. Eat 50 grams of fiber daily.

Do you eat more when you wake up late?

Do you eat more when you are angry?
Do you eat less when you are sick?

Do you eat more when you watch TV or play on your device?

Do you eat only at home or before you go home? This is one of the reasons why it is important to remember that when it comes to healthy living everything is interrelated. Go back to your 72-hour health and wellness audit to check how other factors affect what you eat.

Day 16: Make daily positive sustainable adjustments to your meals

To make sustainable adjustments and modifications to your meals, add variety to what you eat and how you prepare your food. You can begin by asking yourself more questions.

Through the answers to the following questions, you can find your own eating pattern and adjustments that you can make to help you continue eating healthy:

What did you have for breakfast or lunch two days ago? Was it healthy? Was it more plant-based or more processed food?

What about lunch? Was it more processed food? What type of food do you like? What about fruits and vegetables?

What did you eat for supper? When did you eat your cucumber? Did you drink water or soda with your meal?

Did you snack on fruits, cookies, chips, or candy? Do you eat snacks just before you go to bed? How many times do you snack in a day? Is it 3 times a day, 2 times a day or only once? Please write it down.

If you feel full after a meal you may find yourself eating so much food in between meals that you may begin to gain back weight that you may have lost. If you feel hungry between meals, snack small portions of almonds, cashew nuts or peanuts. Almonds will make you feel less hungry and still boost your metabolism, though they take getting used. Have you tried almonds before? Have tired almonds with chocolate?

The challenge is that sometimes even when you know what is right to do or eat, doing it consistently can be a problem. This is part of reason why I always suggest that you have at least 3 to go to nuts that you can rely on, to use as snacks in -between meals. My own go-to nuts are peanuts, almonds, and cashew nuts, all unsalted. What are yours?

How would you cope with any challenges or negativity that your own daily patterns may have revealed?

Do you use food to cope with your daily challenges by drinking alcohol, smoking eating more food or watching porn? This is not a positive sustainable adjustment to your daily meals.

You can make low fat yogurt and chia seeds for your breakfast. Have eggs, nuts, and red meat occasionally. By occasionally, I mean about 2 times a week. Eat fish at least two times a week. How many times do you eat fish every week?

You can further reduce your fat intake by eating skinless chicken or turkey. Turkey and chicken have their fat on their skin, but red meat has most of its fat contained within the meat. Grilling is better than frying.

Always aim to use unsaturated oils like corn, and olive oils for cooking. Do you prefer frying to grilling? Why is this even important to consider? Grilling does not add additional fat or calories to your food. Do you prefer frying to grilling? Why is this even important to consider? It is important because of the relationship between Advanced glycation end products(AGEs) our health, and how food is prepared. According to the NIH, most modern food and related meals are made by heating food , leading to dietary AGEs that contribute to oxidant cellular damage and chronic inflammation that contribute to heart and vascular disease and metabolic disorders like diabetes. AGEs bind to cell surfaces and body proteins affecting cellular and organ function.

Foods rich in protein and fat contain more AGEs than those rich in carbohydrates such as fruits, vegetables, and whole grains. Foods fried tend to have more AGEs than food that is grilled. Part of the reason is that fried food tends to have more fat added as part of the process of preparing the food through frying.

You can also gradually reduce the fat content in your milk products. You can do this by changing the variety of milk that you drink from whole milk to 2% fat: then to 1% fat. I am wary of fat free milk because it is still important to get fat in your body which can be used through cellular metabolism to produce cell membranes and hormones. Choose lower-fat cheese and yogurt. When you buy yogurt, also check that it does not contain sugar. The good thing about reducing to 1% fat milk is that it remains tasty. Fat has 9 calories of energy per gram compared to carbohydrates and proteins that have about 4 per gram.

The main thing in positive sustainability of your meals is to keep in mind that just because you do not have high blood pressure, diabetes, or any other leading cause of death that you know of, does not mean that you are fine, and you don't have to do anything to worry about. You must remain vigilant.

Write down the commonest adjustments you make to your food very day? How many times did you make those adjustments in the past 7 days? Challenge yourself to make positive consistent positive food adjustments in the next 30 days.

Day 17: Make variety part of your daily healthy eating habit.

Make variety part of your daily eating habit. If you plan your meals and snacks ahead of time you will have to make them the variety that will help you to stay heathy and counter the effects of oxidants and chronic inflammation on your body. Take time to plan at least one lunch and dinner every week without meat or cheese and eat more fruits and vegetables.

Get healthy food recipes so that you can either cook healthy food that you will really enjoy or ask someone to help you. Create your meals around whole grains, vegetables, and beans to increase fiber and reduce fat. If you want to have something to chew on, get some fish or tofu. You can make every Friday your fish meal day to begin with then gradually add more and more fish to your meals.

Have at least five servings of fruit and vegetables every day. Choose fruit that is in season. Take an apple per meal. The red delicious apples contain pectin, a fiber that helps to promote healthy cholesterol levels and contain more amounts of antioxidants than many other types of apples.

Do you eat cucumbers every day? Make them part of your daily meal. According to the USDA cucumbers on average contain about 2.8mg sodium and about 193mg of potassium, Vitamin K, Lutein and Zeaxanthin , Ig of fiber and cucurbitacin. Research has shown that cucurbitacin's help to fight liver, breast, lung, and prostate cancer by helping to stop cancer cells from multiplying or growing. On the other hand, the high potassium and very low sodium content of cucumber helps it to reduce blood pressure. Potassium generally helps to lower blood pressure because of its effect on blood vessels and how it counteracts the effect of sodium.

Overall, you can see that eating at least one cucumber per meal would mean that you will be eating a fruit that can help you have cellular and vascular changes that can affect your health and your ability to possibly ward off chronic conditions like cancer and high blood pressure which are some of leading causes of death for those 50 years old and above.

Based on your 72 – hour health and wellness audit, how many servings of fruits and vegetables do you eat in a week? Is it 15 servings per week, based on 3 servings per day? To increase your intake of fruits and vegetables, start by eating every meal with salads consisting of cabbage, tomatoes, carrots, broccoli, bananas, and spinach. Eating a colorful variety of vegetables and fruits per meal with quinoas or reduced portions of brown rice or complex carbs like oatmeal or kinos will make your meal significantly more healthy and bulkier but less energy dense. It will help you to lose significant pounds and keep them off. spinach, tomatoes, cabbage, asparagus, tomatoes, cabbage, and avocado.

During this compass 30-day challenge for longevity make eating one cucumber everyday one of your 30-day challenge habit tracker. At the end of this 30-day challenge your goal would be to be eating more plant - based food per day, and at least 50 g of fiber per day.

Here are a few more tips on what you can do to help you live a healthier and longer life.

*Drink low-fat milk or eat low fat yoghurt with chia seeds.

*Eat at one least one cucumber per day.

*Eat at least five servings of fruits and vegetables daily.

*Eat your food in one location without TV or without your smart phone.

*Eat fish and skinless poultry like chicken or turkey at least once a week.

*Eat only 80% of your meal

*keep to the healthy-eating blue print you have developed , at least 80 percent of the time

*Keep eating right even after a lapse.

What is your 30-day challenge goal for eating with variety? How many times did you add fruits and vegetables to your meal? Do you do that 80 percent of the time? Did you drink water before every meal? Assess your first week and see if you are at least 80 percent closer to the mark you set for yourself, then become more consistent towards the end of your 30-day challenge.

Day 18: Strive to maintain a healthy weight

Day -18, the idea is to help you focus on weight as a way of holding yourself accountable for consistently doing the things you learned so far in this compass longevity challenge. By the time you cut down your food portion, do intermittent fasting, make healthy food choices by eating less processed food and more plant-based food, you probably find yourself weighing less.

Do you weigh yourself every week? If you weigh yourself every week, it will help you keep your weight healthy by keeping better track of your weight or changes to your weight. This way you can catch negative trends early and begin to make changes early.

Weigh yourself before you start then weigh yourself after every week. You can use a simple scale to weigh yourself. Measuring your weight regularly is one of the easiest checks on how your individualized health plan is working. It is easier to do than calculating your BMI. Just climb on a scale and read your weight.

Get a weight-loss journal or notebook. Unless you have a way to regularly evaluate your progress throughout your health and wellness loss journey, you will find sustainable success more difficult to maintain. How can you tell if you are meeting your daily mini goals if you don't evaluate yourself? Evaluating yourself regularly and taking daily positive action will help you form the right healthy habits.

The more you know about how unhealthy food choices can affect your weight, cellular and vascular health, the more you will be interested in making sustainable lifestyle changes. Do you regularly eat your variety vegetables and fruits? If you truly want to maintain a healthy weight you have to eat more plant-based food.

SIMPLE WEIGHT TRACKER

DATE	TIME	WEIGHT	NOTES / COMMENTS

Remember that it is easier to watch your portion and reduce 100 calories food intake, than it is to exercise and burn off the 100 calories that you have eaten. Do you still exercise regularly or have discovered that "you don't have time"? Are you becoming better at managing stress that could arise out of your interactions, conversations, and relationships with yourself and others?

To lose weight and keep it off you track yourself to show whether what you are doing is working or not. You can do this by doing two simple things once a week. Weigh yourself at least once a week and calculate your BMI every three months. Measure your waist circumference once a week. You can also use less formal ways like dress size, change in belt hole, pant size, loose ring, or changes in shoe fitting to evaluate your weight loss journey. Take time to fill in your compass healthy living logbook or journal every day or at least once a week.

This will give you an idea of some factors contributing to your weight gain or stubborn weight loss. Maybe you are spending too much time watching TV or on social media. According to Cleland, Schmidt, Dwyer, &Venn, the (2008) time spent in behaviors that involve a lot of sitting with little activity, like watching or viewing TV was thought to be one of the factors responsible for increasing number of people that are either overweight or obese in different parts of the world. The study also found that in both men and women the average time spent watching television increased with the increasing frequency of consuming food and drinks while watching television. Soft drink consumption during television viewing was associated with a greater increase in abdominal obesity in both men and women.

If on the other hand you discover that you have gained back some of the weight you have lost, then do a quick 72 –hour food audit to see the eating patterns that are making you gain weight. Short-term weight gains usually are as a result of increasing calorie intake or eating more food, rather than simply from reducing physical activity.

Remember that a lapse is not a relapse. A mistake is not a failure. Don't be too harsh on yourself ! If you find yourself not sticking to the eating patterns that can help you eat more fruits and vegetables, try to find out why before making drastic changes.

Do you know that the kind of self-talk you give yourself can affect your weight? This is part of the process of autosuggestion with which you can direct your subconscious mind. If you tell yourself that you can't lose weight, then you will find a way to gain weight even after you have started losing weight or started making the right adjustments. Try again if you do not succeed the first time.

Do not forget to talk to your doctor or health care provider about your medications. Make sure you are not taking any medications or have any underlying disorders that may make you gain weight. This is particularly important if through a chart of your weekly weight measurement you discover that you have gained weight.

Check your list of activities you consider realistic for you to accomplish your weight loss in a day based on your knowledge, experience, personality, available resources, and your stress management skills. Once you have a concrete list in front of you, it's a lot easier to check on yourself regularly and know what lifestyle changes you will need to make.

Remember that maintaining a healthy weight is part of the telomeric lifestyle. Weigh yourself and calculate your BMI. If you can't do it, see your doctor or provider. A combination of exercise, eating healthy and managing stress with good self-care will help lose weight in a realistic and sustainable way.

Remember to weigh yourself today. Make sure you weigh yourself at least every 3 days, in this compass 30-day longevity challenge.

Day 19: Form the habit of effectively managing stress every day

When it comes to managing stress everyday you have to remember that any one of your daily interactions can become a stressor because it can alter the balance or homeostasis within your body system. After all, stress can be defined as a threat to your homeostasis or inner balance caused by a variety of stressors, such as environmental, psychological, or physiological factors (Chung, 2005).

Why is managing stress important for living a healthier and longer life?

Research shows that stress increases the risk of diabetes mellitus, can lead to build up of plaque in arteries(atherosclerosis), especially if combined with unhealthy eating and a sedentary lifestyle, and can lead to anxiety, depression, and severe broncho-constriction in asthmatics (Salleh, 2008).

How does stress affect your cellular and vascular health or your ability to live a healthier and longer life?

Stress affects cellular and vascular health by causing increased mitochondrial activity and increased damaging and shortening of. telomeres. Damaged and shortened telomeres are associated with chronic inflammation and age-related degenerative diseases(Lin and Epel, 2022).

Why should you care about the effect of stress on the length of telomeres? Research found that those 60 years and above with shorter telomere length had earlier all-cause mortality from infectious disease and heart disease (Lin and Epel, 2022).

Stress can affect cellular health by leading to damage to your mitochondria and repeated acute stress in our cells can lead to degenerative diseases, cardiovascular diseases, malignancies, and contribute to the process of aging (Poljšak and Milisav, 2012 ; Chung, 2005).

Research also shows that emotional stress contributes significantly to cancer, cardiovascular disease, accidental injuries, respiratory disorders, liver cirrhosis, and suicide, which are among the leading causes of death in the United States (Salleh,2008). Are you mentally focused enough to maintain your peace of mind and protect your health every day?

First do your do your own 72-hour stress audit so that you can find the most common stressors you have to deal with. You can do this by simply writing down the situations and circumstances that led to stress for you in the past 72 hours.

Write down the common causes of stress in your life based on the audit you did. Were they conversational or non-conversational stressors?

How can you stay calm under pressure?

Daily stress could be from the following:

Conversations

Relationships

One of the biggest sources of stress in your daily life is from your relationships. It may simply be your relationship with your family, friends, or coworkers. One way to reduce this possibility is to ask questions. Asking ourselves these questions and answering them honestly will enable us to enjoy our relationships more fully.

Is someone close to you always telling you that you are not smart enough?

Do you believe them?

Remember that once a person feels hurt through your interaction that person will try to hurt you, no matter how innocent your intention may have been. It does not matter if that person is your spouse, your child, your best friend, your co-worker, your brother, your sister, your patient, client, customer, a stranger or even your boss!

The best way to manage stress from your relationships is to manage your expectations. Lower your expectations in terms of being treated fairly, being understood or appreciated.

Criticisms

Personal expenses

Are you dealing with stress that comes from financial strain?

Your salary is not enough to cover your personal expenses?

You don't have enough money for your spouse to spend?

Work

Are you dealing with a toxic work environment, home environment or social environment?

If you closely analyze the common sources of stress in your life you will discover that 20% of the causes or 1 out of 5 of the common causes of stress will be responsible for 80 % of the stress that you will deal with every day.

What did you find out when you did your analysis? Was 80% of your daily stress from your relationships, conversations, work or money related?

How do you manage stress that arises from minor incidents or conversations?
How do you manage conversational stress??

When dealing with conversational stress think before you speak. It is wise sometimes to think about both a positive or negative response before you ask a question or begin a conversation.

This is not always easy because sometimes what others will say to you will pierce your heart before you know it. It is ultimately your way of reacting to stress that will determine your susceptibility to illness and your overall health and wellness (Salleh,2008).

How do you deal with daily hassles such as arguments at work, at home, or at events, annoying drivers, marital problems, financial difficulties, and challenges at work which could be sources of repeated acute stress or sources of chronic stress?

Focus on what you can control and don't forget the integrative link between your mind, body, and spirit. You can use mind over matter to manage stress. **According to Marcus Aurelius, "A real man doesn't give way to anger and discontent, ….. The nearer a man can come to a calm mind, the closer he is to strength."**

How can you stay calm under pressure?

Learn to look at your conversations with others as a chess game. Don't just talk to others without being mentally prepared for how they would respond to you. This could be a negative response from a person that sees problems in everything you do. With others, it could be a positive response. Remember that if you want to win a chess game, you must be able to anticipate 2 or 3 moves your opponent might make after you have made your first move. When you are talking to others, you must form the habit of anticipating 2 or 3 responses ahead.

In addition to managing conversational stress, do you also manage non-conversational stress. **You can manage non-conversational stress by doing the following:**

- Lower expectations
- Check strategic outcomes/ possibilities
- Step by step do the possible based on your resources, context and time
- Use positive self-talk to help yourself while moving from where you are to where you want to be.

How consistently have you anticipated your responses to others in the past 7 days? In the next 30 days write down the circumstances that led to the most challenging encounters you had with others.

Day 20 : Don't allow daily criticisms make your day negative

How can you manage stress from criticisms?

Expect that no matter how well you do, someone else you find a way to criticize you. Always stay prepared. Remember the following:

Lower your expectations

See problems are gifts

See challenges are opportunities

See criticisms are tests

First stay always stay prepared for daily criticisms. **The more you try to be the best version of yourself by doing the best you can, even in the most challenging or hostile circumstances in your life or**

workplace, the more you shall be challenged to give more or criticized for not doing enough, if you are not doing what others expected or if you are not doing what others like.

For most people, criticisms are one of the audiovisual triggers for stress generation. How can you overcome this tendency? How you react to criticism depends in large part on how you perceive or see criticisms.

Research has shown that criticism can make the one being criticized mentally exhausted, have low esteem, lose confidence, get depressed, anxious, and become more prone to self-harm. The more you are criticized, the more you are likely to want to resist or want to do anything at all. However, if you learn to start looking at criticisms as tests, you can ask yourself which part of yourself is being tested now. Is it your patience, your knowledge, fortitude or self-mastery?

Unless you are prepared to acknowledge that every day of your life you will be

---

criticized by others with little or no recognition of your positive attributes, if they are not happy with what you are doing, you will not be able to have the thoughts for positive personal transformation. Remember that through your thoughts and actions you can influence how your brain responds to your critics.

Remember that you are just as imperfect as the person criticizing you. You are not the sum of your imperfections. You're a complex human being with strengths and weaknesses. Sometimes taking action to protect yourself against criticism would entail giving yourself positive self-talk, at other times it would entail speaking less and listening more!

One way to manage criticisms better is to listen with your senses. How do you do that? Listen with your senses. We must learn to listen without speaking back immediately. Lower your expectations from others when they speak with you.
We have to actively listen with our eyes, ears and even hands. If your hands touch

and it is quickly withdrawn, something is wrong. If a hug is rejected something is wrong. A rising and loud voice suggests the buildup of tension. If deliberate avoidance begins to happen, especially if in the past eye contact was freely made, then something is amiss. Ask questions. Make sure you really heard what you think you heard before you speak.

Keep in mind that there may be other factors or other concerns, others may have that affect their dealings with you or could influence their response to you. There could be hidden antagonistic conversational messages in your interactions with others.

How can use listening with your senses to manage criticisms in your own compass 30-day challenge for longevity? How many times did you keep quiet when you were criticized in the past 7 days? Your goal is to keep quiet and think before you speak or act every day so that by the time you get to the 30th day of your 30-day compass longevity challenge, you have mastered managing daily criticisms.

You can use ideas and strategies below while managing daily criticisms during your 30-day compass longevity challenge.

You can manage daily criticisms by doing the following:

- Lower expectations
- Listen with your senses
- Have conversational chess
- Use positive self-talk to help you anticipate, adjust and become better every day.

Day 21: Challenge yourself to reduce your compass stress index(CSI)

The challenge for day 21, is to reduce your compass stress index(CSI).How manty times do you get into stressful outbursts to the level of losing it in a day? Make a note of the number of times your emotional sense of well-being has been disrupted and you felt stressed out enough to have an outburst during the day. Do this in the morning, the middle of your day and at the end of your day.

If you get into stressful outbursts 10 or more times a week , then your compass stress index is 100 or more or severe. When it is 5 times to 9 times week, your compass stress index is 50 to 90. When it is 2 to 4 times per week, Your Compass Stress Index will be 20 to 40. When your stressful outburst is 0 or once per week, your CSI will be 0 or 10.

Your daily objective would be to keep your Compass Stress Index (CSI) to zero per day or one per week, giving a CSI of not more than 10 per week. This means having 1 or less challenging stressful event per week should be your goal.

At the end of this 30-day compass longevity challenge, you would be able to reduce your baseline compass stress index to less than half of what you started with. You will get to a point where every emotional tension will not lead to a stressful outburst, because you are now more consistently able to use your positive self-talk, chess conversations or simply listening with your senses to manage stress better!

Here is your modified compass stress index(CSI):

Good Compass stress index: 0 to 1 stress outburst per week

Mild Compass stress index: 2 to 4 stress outbursts per week

Moderate Compass stress index:5 to 9 stress outbursts per week (examples include lashing out at others, cutting others off, insisting on your point of view)

Severe Compass stress index: 10 or more stress outbursts per week (This will include pointing at others, speaking with raised voices or being in people's personal space without touching them)

Extreme Compass stress index: Any compass stress index with any hostile contact.

A compass stress outburst is characterized by non-contact emotional disruption that includes anger, confusion, more silence than usual, yelling, disruptive behavior like tension muscles, pounding or striking things without contact with another person.

Hostile contact with another person in terms angrily touching at others, shoving, pushing, fighting, or using or brandishing weapons like knives, guns, sticks, stones, glass, regardless of frequency of daily stressful

---

outbursts is an automatic extreme compass stress index that would require immediate action to diffuse the tension and protect your life.

Why? **Extreme compass stress index means DANGER.** What actions will you take when your house is on fire? Get out of the house as fast as you can and as safely as you can. Do the same when you are dealing or interacting with someone whose behavior has been classified or found to be dangerous or extreme compass stress index. Get yourself out of the situation or get yourself out of their way. Stay vigilant. **Even the most beautiful butterfly still gets eaten by a bird!**

Write down your average compass stress index for the week. The lower the number the better. You should strive for a weekly compass stress index of 10 or less or preferably a daily CSI of zero. What is your daily CSI? Review it after week to your trend. Is it going up or going down?

Get a stress-free -living journal or notebook and take notes of the time and circumstances that typically lead to a stress outburst. This will help you discover your own tendencies, patterns, and the commonest causes of stress for you.

After you have determined or discovered the easy activities that will consistently help you to eliminate and manage stress, take realistic action to transform yourself and get the results you want for yourself. Your goals should be achievable and make sense within the parameters of your life. This includes your health, finances, relationships, family, job, education, spirituality, circumstances, situation, thoughts and actions. Be patient with yourself. Be prepared to learn from your own mistakes or from your critics. Don't expect everyone to like or find no fault in what you are doing,

Don't assume that because you are now a little bit older others will be more accommodating towards you. Always stay prepared for the unexpected. Don't assume that because you have spent most of your life taking care of your spouse, children, and parents, that as you begin to get older, one of them will be there for you or that they won't tell you off!

Check your list of activities you consider realistic for you to accomplish your stress-free living daily objectives in a day based on your knowledge, experience, personality, available resources, and your time – management skills. Once you have a concrete list in front of you, it's a lot easier to check on yourself regularly. You have to stick to your plan and accomplish the tasks on your list one after the other. If you do this day in, day out, week after week, you will gain in your ability manage both the expected and unexpected emotional disruptions and stressful encounters without losing it back! Do you have the discipline to do your best with what you have every day?

Don't let regular evaluation discourage you, instead use it as a tool to discover either new sources of emotional tension or new wrinkles to old sources of emotional tension, so that you can more effectively manage them and protect your health, sense of well-being and happiness.

What is your 30-day stress management challenge? Write down the most common factors or situations that caused you stress in the past 7 days. What is your biggest challenge or area of frustration or anxiety? What are the most common factors affecting your stress status in the past 7 days? What is your compass stress index(CSI)? Did you reduce your CSI by at least 80% at the end of the 30-day challenge?

Day 22: Have more supportive and positive relationships in your life

Do you know that having more supportive and positive relationships will help you live a longer life?

Why are positive and supportive relationships important for living a longer and healthier life? An 85-year Harvard longitudinal research study found that the single most consistent factor for living a longer and healthier life was having positive relationships.

Do you know that you cannot keep positive connections in your relationships without your own daily positive emotional well-being? How can you learn to make the decision to have positive emotional wellness every day? You have to begin by doing a 72- hour relationship audit, to find out the common factors that make your relationships less supportive and positive.

Why does lack of positive and supportive relationships affect our longevity so much? According to the NIH, research has shown that relationship deficits such as

social isolation,

lack of support,

or high strain,

can lead to chronic stress and inflammation, which can be bad for your overall health.

A high strain relationship is full of conflicts, disagreements and lack of common goals and value-adding projects.

Becoming better at managing relationship deficits like lack of support, social isolation and high strain is part of how you can have more supportive and positive relationships.

Research has shown that poorly managed negative emotions can lead to chronic inflammation which can affect your cellular and vascular health and even your brain health, heart health, liver, kidney, and other organs in your body.

What are the most challenging interactions you have had in your relationships?

Is it dealing with problems that arise as part of your daily interaction with those you live with or interact with every day?

Is it dealing with complaints?

Is it dealing with criticisms?

Is it having conversations?

Is it asking questions?

Is it sharing your own point of view?

Every rose has its thorn. Relationships are complex and always involve the plain and hidden. The irritating and the fulfilling. The joy and the pain. They always include positive and negative emotions. You need to develop strategies and habits that will help you have a daily experience more positive emotions than negative emotions in your relationships. Research has shown that those with more positive emotions than negative ones are more resilient and more likely to manage stress better(Fredrickson et al, 2003).

You have to remember that 80% of your disruptions will come from 20% of your encounters?

Reduce your list to the 5 most common encounters with disruptions. Do you know the 1 out of 5 encounters that cause the most disruption to your positive and supportive relationships? How can you always maintain positive interactions in your relationship with others? The key to maintaining positive and supportive relationships in your interactions with others at all times is always to stay prepared for the unexpected. Learn to look at problems or unexpected outbursts, comments or disagreements as opportunities for a more positive navigation in your relationships.

Make the decision not to let the negative things people will say about you when things don't go as expected or they as expected or wanted to pull down your spirit or make you see yourself in negative manner. Accept your mistake or that could have done things better or differently and focus on developing a more holistic process that would help deal with the same event, similar project, encounter or circumstance better. You can't go back to yesterday, but you can learn from what happened to live today more positively.

What are key elements in positive relationships?

Understanding

Value Adding

Respect

Bearing with one another

Forgiveness

Mutual Trust

Do you have trust-related issues in your life? Some people have difficulty trusting others. Some people are more resentful than others when they don't receive the level of trust, they think they deserve or the praise they think deserve in their relationships. While the urge to cheat may be real, you have to remember that once you cheat you destroy trust in your relationship.

Without trust your relationship becomes unhealthy and filled with doubt, stress, and anxiety. Dealing with stress and anxiety every day will make you more prone to chronic inflammation and the related chronic diseases like high blood pressure, auto immune disease, depression, and inflammatory bowel disease.

How do you know that your spouse is really working late when he says he is working late? How do you know that a business trip to New York was not really been a weekend gateway with a lover in Hawaii? Cheating is the result of short-term thinking and will destroy your health and well-being unless you keep your eye on the long-term benefits of a healthy relationship.

Other elements of a positive relationship include the following:

Respect

Bearing with one another

Forgiveness

Why is forgiveness an important part of a positive and supportive relationship? When you forgive others, you let go of the tension that builds up within you when others annoy you, and let go of the stress, anxiety and resentment that could disrupt your internal milieu. Forgiving is like opening a clinched fist, it helps you to become more receptive to others and to see more possibilities.

The more we are able to forgive without being naïve as we get older, the more inner peace and tranquility we shall enjoy as we get older.

Value adding

Making the relationships in your daily life positive is also a decision and a commitment to better communication. You have to make the decision to make your relationships more positive. You have to remember that most relationships are based on what people can get out of it. Keep in mind that most relationships are transactional.

Positive relationships are value-adding relationships. What value do your daily relationships add to your life? What value does person A add to your life? Does your spouse, brother, sister, uncle, auntie add a positive value to your life? Remember that no single person can completely satisfy the needs of another. *Expect to have no more than 80% of your needs fulfilled by your partner, friend or the person you are talking with.* You'll have to find the other 20% somewhere else. This might be the need to watch horror movies with someone else, have intellectual conversations, talk about shopping, talk about sports or even your spirituality with others with others.

What value do they add to your daily interactions? When you talk to those close to you do you feel appreciated, valued or do you feel unappreciated and manipulated? Do you feel judged? Do you feel that you are all still part of a team or is each person now trying to look out only for their own interest, happiness, or enjoyment? Are you interested in a value-driven relationship while your partner is interested in a benefit-driven relationship? It is difficult to have a positive relationship in a cocoon of negativity.

Another way to make your relationships more positive is to manage your expectations. What are your expectations when you communicate with others? Can you deal with the criticisms and conflicts that are part and parcel of daily communication? If you want to maintain your own peace of mind throughout the day, then you have to be prepared for unmet expectations. Sometimes it will come in the form of others not wanting to talk when you want to talk. Sometimes, it will come in the form of others disagreeing with you or calling you names even when you thought you were doing your best and acting in the best interest of everyone. What will you do?

Hurt begets hurt. If someone feels you have hurt them, they will try to hurt you back. It won't matter much if that person is your son, daughter, mother, father, spouse, best friend or co-worker. You have to remember that as long as the someone feels that what you have done or are doing is not right or fair, that person will get a negative emotional response from you or from whatever you say. That person maybe your son, daughter, mom, father, friend or co-worker. Sometimes the response will be subtle and mild, at other times it will be a moderate or even a severe repudiation of you as a person and what you purportedly stand for or believe in. You might even be mocked or called a hypocrite or failure. If you were already mentally prepared for any outcome, you won't really be too surprised by what others say. To foresee is to rule!

If you are the head of the family, the manager, the lead, the director, or boss, be prepared to be blamed more than others.

Don't assume that others will understand when you explain to them why you are struggling or why things are not quite going as planned. Focus on finding your own peace through a gratitude and positive thinking, rather hoping to be understood and appreciated.

Every relationship has its beautiful moments and challenging moments. This is why it is important to make your emotional expectations realistic. Don't expect others to be kind to you or speak kindly about you when they are upset with you.

According to the NIH, psychoneuroimmunology has found that there is a relationship between negative emotions and inflammation. Chronic inflammation leads to poor long-term health (Renna, 2021). One of the keys to effective self-mastery is the ability to embrace your difficulties and challenges. Instead of trying to completely figure out how you can avoid criticisms by doing everything within your power to become compliant with another person's sense of what is right or wrong, focus on the strategies that will help you convert daily criticisms into stress-free encounters by turning them into opportunities for greater improvement and more healthy living.

Nobody is everything the other person expected. Nobody is perfect!

Avoid the belief that a good relationship is good 100% of the time. It is not true and creates unreasonable expectations. It is like expecting perfection from others when you know that no one is perfect. Expect that challenges will occur and be prepared for them. Your health and wellness depend on it!! Make your expectations more realistic. No one person gives 100 percent all the time. Why is it that even when you do not give 100% all the time you expect 100% from others?

How do you manage financial expectations? Financial issues often lead to relationship challenges. It's easy for the feelings of stress and anxiety to be taken out on your partner. Don't assume that the more

---

money you have, the more others will love you and listen to you. You have to blame someone, right? Don't. Build up a team with your partner to deal with financial challenges and other challenges.

Remember resentment-filled relationship is not a supportive and healthy relationship. You need to learn to identify the common sources of resentment in your relationships and avoid them.

What will you do if resentment builds up from the feeling that only one person is doing most of the work or that things are not fair? It could be the sense that one person is doing most of the chores at home, while the other person is not keeping to an agreed division of labor. Who does the dishes every night? Who cooks every day? Who makes the money for the family? Who makes the decisions in the family?

How can you keep positive relationships at home, work, and social surroundings?

How do you know that your spouse is really working late when he says he is working late? How do you know that a business trip to New York was not really been a weekend gateway with a lover in Hawaii? Cheating is the result of short-term thinking and will destroy your health and wellness unless you keep your eye on the long-term benefits of a healthy relationship.

What are some the ways you can you're your relationships more positive.

Set goals for the future together.

Get out of the house at least once a week.

It could be eating out.

It could be going to the movies.

It could be going to a sporting event together or going for a walk together. yoga class, or bowling.

Did you know that daily criticism is one of the factors that can rob you of your positive emotional wellbeing and positive relationships?

Research has shown that maintaining positive emotions like gratitude, pride, joy, interest, hope, inspiration, and contentment will help you to learn how to overcome the weed of daily criticism in your garden of life.

Once you learn to manage the 20% source of 80% of your daily criticisms, you will find yourself having greater peace of mind and good health.

How would you feel if you find yourself in a situation where you are always being corrected or reminded of your faults and inadequacies without any acknowledgement of your positive attributes or positive contributions to your relationship or interactions with others? Most people find such situations unbearable!

One of the ways you can create more positive and supportive relationships is to help yourself have a positive warrior mindset. Self–assertiveness will help you to support your position with facts while being mindful of the other person's feelings and perspective.

When it comes to daily communications, it is important to pay particular attention to how you relate to your family, friends, and co-workers. Though your family may love you and genuinely want the best for you, family members can be brutally critical of your efforts when the results, they get out of your efforts do need meet their emotional and financial needs.

Use your self-talk to prepare yourself for the unexpected. Stick to your healthy living goals even if they are not universally approved.

If you are not able to do this, you will find yourself constantly having misunderstandings and shouting matches with your friends and loved ones. This will lead to daily anxiety, criticisms, frustrations, and stress that can drain your energy and ultimately diminish your ability to live a healthy, long, and intentional life! your thought process and make your communication more effective.

If you change your way of thinking, you will change your life and overcome the fear of failure which can stop you from trying to be your best all the time. in all your dimensions of wellness. **Celebrate small victories along the way but be prepared for unexpected setbacks.** Having small victories as you pursue your ultimate dream will train you for greater success.

If you do not invest in yourself and in your ability to find out new and better ways to make the most out of your daily opportunities, your dreams and goals will remain illusions to be pursued but never attained. You can avoid such an outcome by learning how to spot opportunities and consistently take positive action to transform your opportunities into accomplishments.

In the past 7 days how many times have you had misunderstandings and shouting matches with others? Hopefully not too many times. Write Do you know that feelings of gratitude can contribute to your positive warrior mindset?

Day 23: Challenge yourself to live with more gratitude every day

Are you living with gratitude? What are you grateful for today? Form the habit of starting and ending each day by stating the 3 things you are most grateful for. This is a very important activity that you must start and do every day. This is a simple life transforming habit that can help you put things in perspective and have peace that no one can take away from you.

Remind yourself of 3 things you are grateful for when the going gets tough. It is challenging to keep an attitude of gratitude when things are not going as expected at home, at work or during your daily interactions with others. This is particularly true if you have tried to be the best version of yourself in all aspects of your life and have fallen short.

This typically leads to frustration and anger, and doubt. When you doubt yourself, you can end up with feelings of ingratitude which could be bad for your health. This is not good because according to Bussing et al, ..feelings of gratitude and awe contribute to positive perceptions and cognitions even in the face of illness and disease.

Research has also shown that higher levels of gratitude are directly linked to better social support and reduction in stress and depression(Wood et al., 2008). Can you form the habit of living with gratitude every day?

The simplest way to do this regularly is to remind yourself of the reasons why you are grateful. You could be grateful that you are healthy and do not have to deal with a life-changing illness that could prevent you from working and earning the livelihood that allows you and your family to live the lifestyle that you have.

You could be grateful for little things in your life like safely driving to work or going to the grocery and coming back safely. As long as you are not dealing with death, you should be grateful that whatever you are dealing with, could have been worse. missing hitting a pedestrian at the crosswalk or having an accident.

Did you know that an attitude of gratitude can help you deal better with situations such as having diabetes, high blood pressure, COPD, heart failure or COVID 19 or financial challenges?

Remind yourself that when you remember the things you are grateful for when the going gets tough will help you to become more positive. It is challenging to keep an attitude of gratitude when things are not

---

going as expected at home, at work or during your daily interactions with others.

You have to learn how to focus on an attitude of gratitude even when you think you are not being treated fairly! This is hard because the natural tendency is to lash out in anger when others annoy you or you get disappointing results.

Are you grateful for challenges? Have you developed your mind or your spirituality to the level where you now see problems as gifts or opportunities to become better.

It is also important to remember that research shows that gratitude has elements of subjective well-being such as lower negative effect, life satisfaction, and higher positive effect and elements of psychosocial or eudaimonic well-being such as purpose in life, personal autonomy, positive relations with others and environmental mastery (Mills et al, 2015).

You have to remember that one of the best ways to keep an attitude of gratitude is to try to work hard at accomplishing your daily tasks. If you stop worrying about outcomes and focus on giving your best effort in every situation you find yourself, you will positively feel more fulfilled and less stressed out.

Gratitude will help you to engender positive emotions which will help you reduce chronic inflammation and improve your health. According to NIH, an attitude of gratitude is associated with better mood and sleep, less fatigue, more self-efficacy, and a lower cellular inflammatory index (Mills et al, 2015).

Do you know that gratitude is one of the ways one of the ways you can manage stress? How can an attitude of gratitude help you to eliminate stress when things go wrong? An attitude of gratitude can help you to eliminate stress in your daily life by helping you change how you think about the situation.

Do you have a gratitude journal? Start your own gratitude journal today, if you don't already have one.

What is your 30-day gratitude challenge?

*List 3 things you are grateful for every day.

*Plant gratitude trees for your birthday. You can plant it for every birthday or plant it for your 50th birthday, 60th, 65th birthday, 70th and so on.

*You can start a gratitude journal that you fill out every weekend.

*You can pray for more gratitude if you are a person of faith, or you can meditate on gratitude.

*Challenge yourself to be grateful for people, conditions, and things.

*Share your sense of gratitude with others and encourage them to share their own sense of gratitude.

Become more consistent in seeing new ways you can find gratitude in your daily life as you get older. Get your guided longevity journal to keep track of things that make you have gratitude and the things that make you have less gratitude. Out of 30 days, did you meet your goals at least 80% of the time.

Day 24: Form the habit of living with a positive warrior mindset

A positive warrior mindset is one of the keys to living a longer life and it is also a key to having a positive outlook in life. Why is a positive mindset one of the keys to living a healthier, longer and happier life?

A study from John Hopkins found that those with family history of heart disease who also had a positive outlook were about 33% less likely to have a heart attack or related cardiovascular event in 5 to 25 years than those who had a negative mindset or outlook. When your mind becomes overwhelmed by negativity you lose the ability to look at things positively. You lose the ability to look at things with a positive warrior mind set.

Write down a list of your activities and actions in the past 72 hours of your life and see the situations and circumstances that

---

predominantly made you look at things negatively or have negative feelings about yourself and your circumstance.

Do you know that communication is an important part of a positive warrior mindset? Do you remember that the "C" in the compass profile represents community relationships and communications? Research shows that supportive communication means a more problem-oriented rather than person-oriented communication.

You have to remember that the way you communicate with yourself will significantly affect the outcome of anything you do. According to Marcus Aurelius, "The happiness of your life depends on the quality of your thoughts." This shows that if you have mainly negative thoughts or a negative pattern of thinking, you will bring a negative quality to your life.

Do you have a negative or positive pattern of thinking? Your negative pattern of thinking can cloud your thoughts and rob you of the clarity that you need to make outcome-driven decisions. Negative thinking can make some people make the wrong decision and drink so much alcohol that they lose control of their mind and end up getting involved in fights, drunk driving, or toxic activities. Sometimes such behavior can lead to the death of innocent bystanders.

One of the factors that can disrupt how you feel about yourself is the type of person you interact with. If you are dealing with someone who is usually quick to judge or very negative in outlook be prepared to bend without breaking during your communication or interaction with them. Don't allow their point of view or actions to make you have a cloud of negativity.

What will you do if someone calls you names or says things like, "you are wicked", you are difficult", "you are always unfair", such words or sentences will make you feel undervalued and unappreciated. When people feel bad about themselves, they tend to strike back in anger. Our emotions or feelings help us to relate to ourselves and to others. Your emotions can be part of how you communicate with others. This is why any change in our emotional well-being can have a very serious impact on our relationships. It can very easily lead to negative interactions.

People don't take negative interactions well because they lead to negative emotions or overall negativity. Does that mean that we should focus on positive things and deny negative emotions? No. You have to remind yourself that one of the keys to healthy living is focusing on what you can control. You can control your ability to try to be the best version of yourself in everything you do, but you cannot control how people will interpret it or react to your efforts.

While it is good to find out why you are not getting the result you expected from your interactions with others, finding out how you can get better results will help you think more clearly and strategize more effectively.

Everyone makes mistakes but only those with a positive warrior mind set learn how to minimize them and get better results, rather than wallowing in explanations and recriminations. You too can have a positive warrior mind set!

The key task of today's challenge is using your positive warrior mindset to overcome those who are more fault-finding towards you, who will tell you that you don't know what you are doing or that you are grossly incompetent. This is part of an evaluative and person-oriented communication that leads to hurt on both sides.

How can you overcome a person-oriented negative communication directed towards you? **You have to focus on getting a positive emotional outcome out of every encounter you have with others.** This is not easy because personal attacks during interactions with loved ones, friends or co-workers can become painful emotional wounds. To deal with these types of negative interactions, outbursts, or attacks, remind yourself that every opinion is not an automatic reflection of the truth.

What is your 30-day longevity positive warrior mind set challenge? Write down at least 3 positive outlook for the day.

Day 25: Stay vigilant during your daily interaction with others

Stay vigilant when talking to others. Understand that differences in opinion, differences in perception of reality, differences in emotional reaction to similar situations and circumstances or even how things can be done, can lead to escalation of negativity. How can you manage the escalation of negativity in your daily interactions with others?

If you have a growth mindset or a positive warrior mindset you will focus on the steps that he or she needs to take every day to help you stay more positive as you deal with the situation and circumstances you find yourself in. Remember that "Your present circumstances don't determine where you can go; they merely determine where you start." Nido Qubein. Remember that a positive mindset can help you find hope even in the most challenging situations and circumstances.

Can you commit yourself to unlimited daily positive action despite numerous challenges and disappointments? Can you commit to consistently taking small positive steps every day? You can do this by developing a growth mindset. According to Carol Dweck, a renowned psychologist, a fixed mindset person believes that his or her basic qualities, like talent and intelligence, are fixed and cannot be improved. A person with a growth mindset believes that qualities like talent and intelligence can be improved. Fixed mindset people believe that talent alone creates success without effort. It is like believing that you are either born great or you are not.

Research has shown that those with a growth mindset make positivity the unifying motivational thread throughout all these changes you deal with every day. Focus more on finding positive solutions in every encounter than on complaining.

How many times in the past 7 days did you complain? How many times did you look for solutions rather than pointing fingers? The more time you spend complaining the less you will get done. Instead of complaining start taking positive action that can lead to the outcome that you would want.

Act on your ideas. Don't let the perfect become the enemy of the possible. If you have a positive warrior mindset, you will have the ability to consistently make the right adjustments when the unexpected happens.

What are the positive adjustments you can make every day ?

*Stop complaining.
*Focus on what you can control

What steps do you need to take every day How many adjustments did you make in the past 7 days that helped you diffuse tension and get more of the positive result you wanted in your relationships, family, with your friends, at work or social events?

Remember that to foresee is to rule. Form the habit of looking at things, situations and even the achieving of your goals from a solutions perspective rather than from a blaming and complaining perspective. A situation that requires a solution can be approached in a variety of ways. Expect the unexpected.

What is your positive warrior mindset 30-day challenge? How many times in the past 7 days did you communicate more positively or look at problems from a solution perspective than from a blame perspective? How many times were you able to neutralize your negative thoughts through positive self-talk in the past 30 days? How many times were able to make positive adjustments when the unexpected happened? You need to get to being able to have more positivity from your interactions at least 80% of the time.

DAY 26: Pay attention to falls and accidents part of your holistic self-care every day

While it is important to improve your health and live longer by doing most of the things that I have shared with so far in this book or training, it is still possible for us to inadvertently cut our lives short by failing to take simple steps that can help us protect our lives through holistic self-care.

Paying attention to your holistic self-care is the eighth key to longevity. Don't ignore your COMPASS physical profile. How can you improve yourself and your self-care today, if you have no idea of how to control the factors that could influence your health?

Are you cautious and careful? What do you think will happen to you if you exercised every day, ate healthy, slept well but didn't pay attention to falls and accidents? This simply shows that you are not paying attention to your holistic self-care. Why is this important? According to research the top three preventable injury-related death in the United States are poisoning, motor vehicles, and falls.

Did you do a periodic gap analysis in your life to discover those areas in your life and environment that need improvement? Are you in a toxic relationship? Are you in a value adding or value subtracting relationship? Are you actively participating in your own health and wellness journey?

A few years ago, there was the tragic story of 78-year-old man in Los Angeles who tragically fell into the pool in his son's house and died. The saddest part of the story was that the son had invited his father over to spend the week there, so that he could spend more time with his grand kids. While this particular fall led to drowning, at other times falls among those 65 years and above have led to hip fractures, broken necks, spinal and head injuries.

*Protect your home from falls and accidents.

Important daily healthcare activities include the following:

Be careful not to fall at home as you ger older.

Be careful not to get into motor vehicle accidents.

Leave with plenty of time to spare because life happens.

Don't drink and drive.

Don't drive when your very angry.

Keep in mind that uncontrolled anger could lead to immediate road rage, deadly fights or shoot outs. Is someone cutting you off worth dying for?

Let go when drivers cut you off

Don't focus so much on eating healthy, walking at least 10,000 steps, and managing stress that ignore basic self-care activities. Part of holistic self-care is paying attention to details. For others the problem is not falls, but motor vehicle accidents. One of the challenges with accidents is that sometimes you may be in a hurry for other reasons then find yourself driving too fast. What if you had started your morning with a drink of fruit smoothies, done your morning exercise and meditation but because you were running late to work or a meeting you forgot to put on your seat belt, and while driving too fast ended up in an accident? Will this be a good outcome for your longer life?

Do you know the most common factors that can affect your holistic self-care? Do your own 72-hour audit to get an idea. Some of the factors that can affect your holistic self-care would include the falls and accidents already mentioned above and other factors that include personal habits and community relationships.

Keep an eye on yourself through the regular use of health and wellness journals or even the appendix in this book that contains the compass profile and other tables, trackers and journals that you can fill up as part of holding yours. anger has to be part of your

Remember every action will lead to a reaction. Learn to take chess actions. Think about two of three reactions before you take your first action, and ask yourself if your first is worth it or not?

Your holistic self-care also involves your environment and how you interact with it. A few years ago, a 27-year-old healthy young woman went to the Grand Canyon, and in attempt to take a selfie, slipped off the edge and fell to her death. This is an example of not paying close attention to your surroundings and environment at all times. Paying attention to your surroundings and your environment is part of your immediate holistic self-care.

Have you formed the habit of paying attention to your surroundings and environment? Don't forget that Brutus betrayed Cesar. Be careful with the kind of friends that you hang out with. Some friends will try get you drunk, poison you or fail to warn you when they see a life-threatening danger coming your way. To foresee is to rule.

Don't ignore going for your yearly physical or doing your recommended screening tests because of your age or family circumstance or history because you are busy or don't really feel like it.

Don't ignore or dismiss nagging or persistent symptoms without proper checkup because this could be the difference between discovering cancer at an early stage or at an advanced stage.

How many times did you fall or have a near fall in the past 7 days? Keep a close eye on physical environment in the next 30 days, starting from today.

.

DAY 27: Make sure you regularly take your daily vitamins and supplements.

Do you know that taking your daily vitamins can be part of daily self-care? Do you know that regularly taking vitamins every day is one of the ways you can improve your self-care? Take your daily supplements but do not let them replace your healthy habits and do not forget to let your physician know that you are taking vitamins and supplements.

Don't assume that simply because you use multivitamins you will remain perfectly healthy or suffer only mild illness. Remember that vitamins are usually supplemental and your taking daily multivitamins will be most effective only if you continue to eat healthy, exercise regularly and continue to manage your weight and the sources of daily stress in your life.

For example, take your omega 3 and 6 fatty acids which have been proven to be very helpful for the heart. However, do not give up on fish just because you take Omega fatty acids. Still stick to the habit of eating fish rich in Omega fatty acids at least once a week.

Make sure you talk to your doctor about any supplements you are taking or plan to take. This is because if there are interactions or potential interactions between your supplements and any medication you are taking your doctor will let you know.

Taking your supplements should not stop you from going for your regular medical checkup as recommended for your age group and family history by your doctor or health care provider.

For example, we know that vitamin B can be found in fish, meat, orange juice and fortified cereals, yet we also know we do not always get to eat enough of the food. If you combine trying to eat right with taking your vitamins, you will end up regularly getting enough vitamin B in your body. This is an example of how you can use vitamins as a health supplement.

Why are B vitamins so important? Because they help to lower the level of homocysteine in blood vessels, which at high levels can lead to damage of the lining of arteries and could lead to a faster formation of blood clots.

How consistently do you take your vitamins every day? How many times did you miss taking your vitamins in the past 7 days? Write down how consistently you took your vitamins in the next 30 days.

DAY 28: Pay particular attention to protecting your brain health and your memory

One easy way to pay particular attention to your brain health and protect your memory is to form the habit of taking vitamins and supplements every day. Keep in mind that vitamins and supplements are not a magic solution part of effective self-care is discussing your health and options with your doctor.

You can begin by taking Omega 3 fatty acids daily. Apart from supporting heart health, Omega 3 is also good for brain health because research has shown that omega-3 fatty acids help to build cell membranes in the brain. You can get Omega 3 fatty acids from supplements or from fish. This is one of the reasons why it is recommended that you eat fish at least once a week. Begin by making the decision to eat fish at least once a week, you will help your brain health and memory as you get older.

Remind yourself that you are trying to protect your brain health and preserve your cognitive functions such as attention, learning, thinking, problem solving, decision making, and memory for as long as you can as you get older. The more you preserve your cognitive functions and memory as you get older, the less mistakes, accidents and falls you are likely to have as you get older.

Eating more fish in your meals will help to get more of the EPA and DHA omega fatty acids that will protect your cells and fight off inflammation and preserve your brain health and the health of your other organs. Keep in mind that it is not a magic wand for all your problems.

Are you getting enough magnesium into your system? How does magnesium affect your health and wellness? Research has shown that magnesium can help to protect your brain health, help you sleep better and lower your blood pressure. What is the best way of getting your daily magnesium?

How much magnesium is recommended daily? For women the recommended daily amount of magnesium is 320 mg and for men, 420mg. A common and easily available source of magnesium is banana. Instead of relying on a single fruit to get your daily magnesium, it may be better to include other foods and fruits like avocado, leafy green vegetables, and nuts like almonds, cashew nuts and peanuts. Other sources of magnesium include chia seeds, pumpkin seeds, brown rice, and black beans.

When you find that you cannot get enough magnesium from your daily meals, consider adding magnesium supplements to what you eat daily. Be careful with supplements because of the potential for magnesium toxicity and make sure you let your doctor know that you are also on supplements. Why should you consider paying more attention to magnesium than you may have done in the past?

Why is magnesium important to your cellular and vascular health? According to the National Institute health, magnesium affects membrane integrity, muscle contraction, hormone secretion and intermediary metabolism. Magnesium also helps in the movement of calcium and potassium across cell membranes, that can affect heart rhythm and nerve conduction.

Why should you take magnesium supplements or eat more almonds, chia seeds or black beans that contain magnesium as part of your way of improving your brain health and memory? Recent research findings have shown that magnesium can help your brain health by helping your brain shrink less with less white matter lesions. Researchers also found that taking magnesium per day as recommended could lead to less risk of memory loss, age-related dementia, and help with keeping our cognitive functions for longer as we get older.

The other two things that you can do that will help protect your brain health and memory will be taking more steps every day and doing more puzzles or doing more activity books weekly. When it comes to puzzles and activity books , do one new book per week. If you are still not doing 10,000 steps a day, on day

Another way to stay mentally active and stay connected to a community is to get a hobby. Develop a noteworthy hobby that you can practice with a group of people in a safe environment. This will help you adjust your work-life balance and lessen or minimize the impact of problems in your daily life. Your hobby could be playing baseball, basketball, golf, dancing, fishing, running, tennis or even playing Sudoku. It could also be any other unique activity that preferably has a mental, spiritual and physical component that you can participate in on a regular basis that would help take your mind away from the activities that typically consume your day.

Do you have a family or personal history of obesity–related illnesses like diabetes, high blood pressure, heart attack or stroke?

If you have a blood pressure cuff, measure your blood pressure today. If you do not have one, go to the nearest pharmacy, and use their free blood pressure cuff to find out your blood pressure. The steps outlined so far are things you can do for yourself now, especially if you feel you are healthy but have not taken any objective steps to check your health for years. Maybe your last health check was in school or when you got hired or just before you retired.

How many puzzle and activity books have you done in the past 7 days? Do you check your health numbers regularly? Make sure you make the checks as already discussed in the next 30days, starting from today.

Day 29: Make sure you are paying attention to managing active-illness and potential long-term problems

What is your self-care strategy for managing active illness? Do you collaborate with your doctors? Do you listen to them, then ask questions and take action that will help you become better? You need to take your medications, do the tests that you are asked to do and go to your appointments. If you are still in doubt or need further assurance about the direction of care or your prognosis, seek a second opinion.

If you have not seen your doctor in a long time set up an appointment with your health care provider to enable you get a more detailed picture of your metabolic profile, especially your cholesterol level, blood sugar, potassium, vitamin D and other tests relevant to your family and medical history.

What are the other important self-care aspects you need to know and do. Do you brush your teeth every morning and night?

Do you ignore your oral health and personal hygiene in your health and wellness journey? **Poor oral health can lead to systemic diseases like heart disease, pneumonia and cancer to name a few.**

Don't forget your eyes. Are you seeing your eye doctor regularly? Do you know that research shows that taking 5 mg of melatonin every night can help your eye health?

When was the last time you saw your doctor? Do you get your immunizations as needed? If you need to get vaccines, get your vaccines like the flu vaccines or COVID 19 vaccines. Do not just say you are eating healthy, exercising, and taking your supplements; therefore, you do not need to get your vaccines. If you need to bundle up because it is cold, do it. Wash your hands frequently to minimize your chances of getting an infection.

Do you also know that focusing on gratitude despite your daily changes can be part of your daily self-care?

An attitude of gratitude will help you deal with daily challenging situations calmly. This will help you to overcome your stress.

Learn to lower expectations during your interactions with others. Lower the expectation that you will be understood or that your own context or perspective will be understood. This will help to have better emotional balance, which is a very important aspect of your emotional wellness and holistic self-care.

What about sociocultural self-care? Are you a value adding person? Do you add value to your culture and community? As you get older people can say that you have contributed positively to your cultural heritage. Do you stay connected to your community?

What about your spiritual self-care? Do what is right for your spirituality without condemning others? Do you do your meditations and regularly go to your faith-based services. Research shows that if you have a lifestyle with spirituality and religion, you have a healthier and longer life!

What is holding you back from improving your health every day? Is it that you are too busy? Is it that you don't have a better self-mastery of yourself? While self-mastery requires more mental energy to set up, once you have achieved greater self-mastery you will require less energy to function more effectively through good positive healthy habits.

Your brain likes to reduce the energy it spends to accomplish tasks, which is part of the reason we form habits. Research has shown that about 40 % to 50% of our daily activities are shaped by habits. Do you know the habits that dominate your own daily activities? Are they good habits or bad habits?

Do you deal with stress by smoking or drinking alcohol? Do you know drinking too much alcohol is not good for your health?

*Don't smoke. If you are still smoking, make plans to stop. Don't use smoking, alcohol and sex as coping mechanisms for managing stress or dealing with challenging or negative relationships.

Consider taking advantage of free informational health exams or blood work offered at your office or your membership clubs or insurance to get your cholesterol or metabolic profile.

*Do you have a family history of high blood pressure, diabetes, cancer, or glaucoma?

*Start each day with meditation and exercise and a plan for the day. Make this part of your compass blue print or process.

*Keep quiet if you have nothing positive to say.

*Become familiar with your family and medical history.

*Review your health insurance regularly.

*Get more education. That will help you become a better health self-advocate

*Stay vigilant in all your interactions with others.

* What area of self -improvement did you focus on in the past 72 hours?

*Forgive yourself and others daily

*Sleep at least seven to eight hours a day.

*Cut down on unnecessary expenses.

*Call a friend today.

*Review your finances monthly

*How much money do you make in a week and how much money do you spend in a week?

*Help at least one person each day.

*Meditate or say a prayer or do both.

*Form a healthy living group of friends and family that you can trust or join one.

*Check your blood pressure weekly.

*Weigh yourself weekly

*Take your multivitamins regularly.

*Is it at night, day, or morning?

*Work for your future everyday
.*Continue to write on journal at least once a week.

.

After the check up, you have to follow through with the labs and tests you have to do. You have to go to the pharmacy and get your medications. After you get your medications, you must take them or make sure you don't mix them up when taking them, if not you will not get the desired result.

Please write down how many times you took your medications in the past 7 days. Use your 30-day tabulation or journal notes, to keep yourself accountable, starting from today.

Day 30: Review what you have done and challenge yourself to use your holistic habits for better daily self-care

Challenge yourself to form habits that will help you review and improve daily. What is the essence of your holistic wellness and healthy living if it will not help you live a happy, healthy, longer, and more positive and fulfilled life?

Do you know the habits that dominate your own daily activities? Are you an early riser? Do you get your projects done right away or at the last minute? Do you like to get things done step by step or on the fly? Do you easily get distracted, or do you begin one project and finish it before you start another?

A habit can be defined or described as a behavior that is recurrent, that is acquired or formed through repeated action that is usually brought on by a cue or social context (Rubin, 2015). Research has shown that about 40 % to 50% of our daily activities are shaped by habits. Have you formed the habits that will help you pursue and achieve your daily goals?

The decision to live a happier, healthier, and longer life has to be supported by daily positive thoughts and actions consistent with holistic habits and your own compass blueprint for healthy living.

What will you do every day to review and improve your health and wellness daily?
Here are examples of the few things you can do regularly as part of daily holistic self-care:

*Start each day with meditation, exercise and a to-do list

*Keep your daily compass stress index(CSI) to one or zero (1 or 0)

*Focus on cutting down unnecessary expenses

*Did you call a friend today as part of positive and supportive relationships?

*Have you helped at least one stranger or someone you didn't know in the past 7 days?

*Write down your feelings and experiences.

*Do check your blood pressure once a week or as often as you have been asked to by your doctor?

*Do you weigh yourself every 3 days or at least once a week?

*Do you take your multivitamins or supplements regularly?

---

*Do you keep your appointment with your healthcare providers?

*Stay vigilant in all your interactions with others.

*Focus on forgiving yourself and others daily

*Don't expect others to forgive you because you apologized or explained your perspective.

*Stick to daily supportive communications

*Keep quiet when you have nothing positive to say

*Sleep at least seven to eight hours a day

*How many times did you reach out to a friend or relative in the past one week?

*What simple steps can you take today to have better health?

*Do you meditate every day?

*Have you formed a healthy living group of friends and family that you can trust or joined one?

*How many hours a day do you spend on social media or on the phone?

*Get a blood pressure logbook and use it.

*Keep your appointment with your healthcare providers.

*Keep eating right even after a lapse.

*When was the last time you did your yearly physical?

*Take care of your oral health, personal hygiene and self-care

*Do you do your screening tests as recommended by your healthcare providers?

*Become familiar with your family and medical history.

*Do you have the most quarrels and conflicts in the morning, afternoon , and evening?

*Have you reviewed your health insurance in the past 30 days?

*Do you put in the time to learn more about the things that are good for your health?

*Do you protect your home from falls and accidents?

*Work for your future everyday
.

*Do you write down your emotional challenges every 3 days?

*Do you say 3 things you are grateful for every day?

*How many hours do you spend watching TV every day?

---

*Do you drink alcohol to cope with stress or deal with your daily challenges?

*Do you like to get things done step by step or on the fly?

Start your own longevity journal with some of the answers to the above questions and related guidance. Start a health and wellness journal. Get pen and paper and write down your own answers to the questions above or type them into your computer, phone, or mobile device. Do some journaling to help you hold yourself more accountable.

Overall, how well have you been keeping up with the mini-challenges from your 30-day longevity challenge? The answers you give to these questions will help find out if you are doing your best to improve your longevity 80% of the time. Keeping to the 80:20 rule through your habits, daily activities, and lifestyle changes will help begin to live a healthier, happier, longer and more fulfilled life as you get older!

Appendix I : The compass profile

What is the Compass Profile? Do you know how the different components of the compass profile can help you do better?

The components of the compass profile are the following:

C= Community Relationships or Communication profile.
O = Operational capacity profile.
M= Metabolic profile.
P= Physical profile.
A= Ambition profile.
S= Spiritual profile.
S = Self Knowledge profile.

The COMAPASS METHOD is the holistic approach to continuous self-improvement and transformation in health, wellness, and self-mastery based on using the compass profiles and specific compass guidelines.

Understanding and applying the different compass profiles to your situation and circumstances will help you become better at dealing with the root cause of the factors affecting your longevity.

The community relationships profile is essentially your communications profile. The way you communicate and relate with yourself and with others will affect whether you will have value- adding relationships or not. Do you know what is affecting your confidence in yourself and your ability to make effective decisions? Is it fear of the process or fear of communication with others? Is it fear of failure? Communicate with yourself first and write down your deepest fears and worries. Is it what others will say?

Ask yourself questions that will help you recognize which aspects of your relationship with others could either be contributing to your failure to build positive and supportive relationships or could be making things worse. Remember that when you are communicating with others, they will interact with you from their own perspective, worldview, personality, or experience.

Lower your expectations that others will understand you or see things from your perspective. Don't let others frustrate you or disrupt your focus on meeting your 30 -day challenge for living longer.

What is your operational capacity profile? Your operational capacity is your ability to get things done or to make adjustments when the going gets tough and still get things done. Minimize excuses and explanations. The key is that you need to know your limitations or challenges and how to navigate through them. What resources do you have to support or help you as you continue to try to do the specific 30-day compass challenge that you have to do?

Do you know how to look at problems as gifts, and challenges as opportunities? Try to reduce complex problems to small segments that you can accomplish. Begin where you are, not where you want to be. Step by step do the possible.

Do you know your metabolic profile? This is a way of looking at yourself at the micro level. When was the last time you got your blood work done? Your **metabolic profile** will include both your nutritional and metabolic analysis. You can get your metabolic analysis by getting your appropriate physiological and laboratory tests done. help. Getting the right tests done with the help of a healthcare professional or your doctor will make it easy for you to know which aspect of your health you need to focus on improving.

The Physical Profile includes your weight, height, waist circumference, BMI (Body Mass Index) and your environment. It also includes your heart rate and lung function. Movement and structures in your body are a big part of your physical profile. Make sure you exercise every day in a safe environment so that avoid falls and exposure to avoidable harm. Keep it simple and moderate , if you want something more vigorous check with your doctor before you begin. After all, checking with your doctor or getting additional information from an expert is a very important part of self-care.

The fifth compass profile is your ambition profile. You can use your ambition profile to assess your drive and motivation. What motivates you? What are your goals? Are you motivated more by the thoughts of success, or fear of failure? You can use the ambition profile to set **measurable goals like walking at least 10,000 steps a day or eating at least 50 g of fiber every day.** Are you motivated enough to achieve your goals through determination and commitment? **Don't quit at the first obstacle.**

The remaining two profiles are **Spirituality and Self Knowledge profiles. The compass spirituality profile focuses on your** relationship with yourself, others, your community, the universe or with God, if you are a person of faith. Do you have a sense of connection to a higher power or does a purpose beyond yourself or your own benefits drive your thoughts, meditations and actions? How can you apply your own spiritual profile to the 30-day compass longevity challenge? A better understanding of your sense of self will help you develop your own positive warrior mindset in a way that will work for you.

The seventh compass profile is your self-knowledge life. Do you know if you have predominantly positive thinking or negative thinking? Do you know your **personality, personality** traits or tendencies, character and mindset? Do you have self-mastery?

A better understanding of your psychosocial strengths and weaknesses will help you know your limitations, and your tendencies, when it comes to forming holistic habits and taking simple steps that will help you live a healthier and longer life.

You can use the 7 components of the compass profile to develop a more holistic approach to living longer.

Appendix II: Tables, trackers and journals

TABLE 1A

Day	Number Of Steps	Minutes of walking	Jump Rope skips	Number of Push ups	Number of distractions
1					
2					
3					
4					
5					
6					
7					
8					
9					
10					
11					
12					
13					
14					
15					

.TABLE 1B

Day	Number Of Steps	Minutes of walking	Jump Rope skips	Number of Push ups	Number of distractions
16					
17					
18					
19					
20					
21					
22					
23					
24					
25					
26					
27					
28					
29					
30					

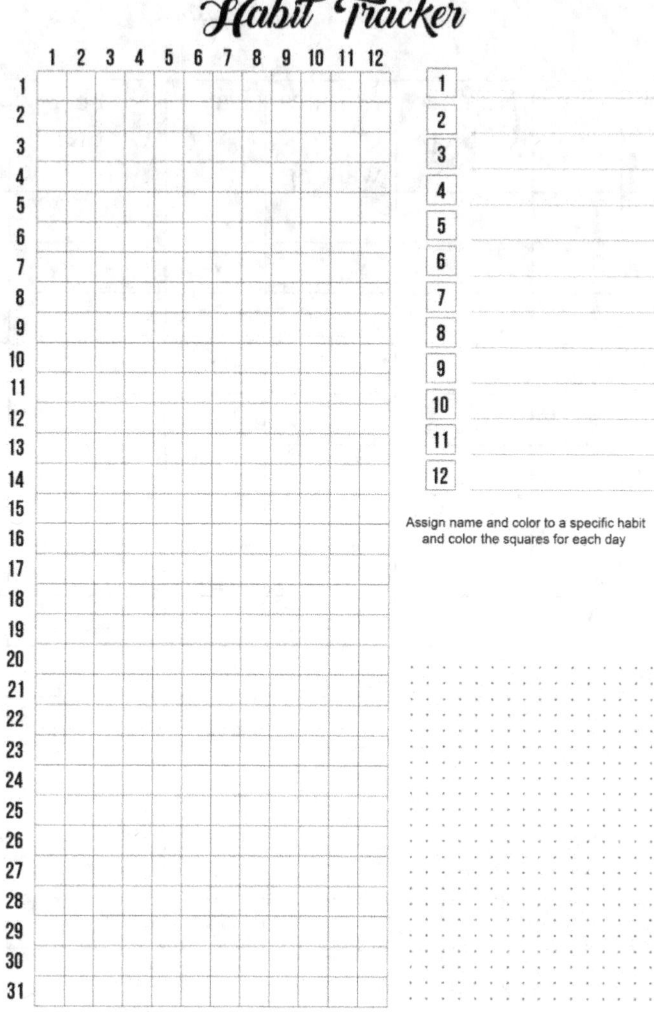
Habit Tracker
1 2 3 4 5 6 7 8 9 10 11 12
1
2
3
4
5
6
7
8
9
10
11
12
13
14
15
16
17
18
19
20
21
22
23
24
25
26
27
28
29
30
31
1
2
3
4
5
6
7
8
9
10
11
12
Assign name and color to a specific habit
and color the squares for each day

TABLE 2

Day	Number Of Steps	Minutes of walking	Day	Number Of Steps	Minutes Of walking
1			16		
2			17		
3			18		
4			19		
5			20		
6			21		
7			22		
8			23		
9			24		
10			25		
11			26		
12			27		
13			28		
14			29		
15			30		

TABLE 3A

Day	Number Of Steps	Hours on TV	Number of Distractions	Hours of Sleep
1				
2				
3				
4				
5				
6				
7				
8				
9				
10				
11				
12				
13				
14				
15				

TABLE 3B

Day	Number Of Steps	Hours on TV	Number of Distractions	Hours of Sleep
16				
17				
18				
19				
20				
21				
22				
23				
24				
25				
26				
27				
28				
29				
30				

TABLE 4A

Day	How many times did you wake up at night? day	How many times did go to bed with device in your hand?	Number of Dreams	Hours of Sleep
2				
3				
4				
5				
6				
7				
8				
9				
10				
11				
12				
13				
14				
15				

TABLE 4B

Day	How many times did you wake up at night? day	How many times did go to bed with device in your hand?	Number of Dreams	Hours of Sleep
16				
17				
18				
19				
20				
21				
22				
23				
24				
25				
26				
27				
28				
29				
30				

TABLE 4C

Day	Did you travel?	What time did you come back from work?	What time did you eat before sleeping?	Hours of Sleep
1				
2				
3				
4				
5				
6				
7				
8				
9				
10				
11				
12				
13				
14				
15				

TABLE 4D

Day	Did you travel?	What time did you come back from work?	What time did you eat before sleeping?	Hours of Sleep
16				
17				
18				
19				
20				
21				
22				
23				
24				
25				
26				
27				
28				
29				
30				

TABLE 5

Day	Blood Pressure	Day	Blood Pressure	Comments
1		16		
2		17		
3		18		
4		19		
5		20		
6		21		
7		22		
8		23		
9		24		
10		25		
11		26		
12		27		
13		28		
14		29		
15		30		

SIMPLE WEIGHT TRACKER

DATE	TIME	WEIGHT	NOTES / COMMENTS

TABLE 6A

Day	Number Of Steps	Average daily grams of fiber	Number of servings of fruits and Veggies	Compass Stress Index (CSI)
1				
2				
3				
4				
5				
6				
7				
8				
9				
10				
11				
12				
13				
14				
15				

TABLE 6B

Day	Number Of Steps	Average daily grams of fiber	Number of servings of fruits and Veggies	Compass Stress Index (CSI)
16				
17				
18				
19				
20				
21				
22				
23				
24				
25				
26				
27				
28				
29				
30				

12 COMPASS LONGEVITY GUIDELINES

Do you?	1	2	3	4	5	6	7	8	9	10
Meditate on 3 things you are grateful for every day										
Do 10,000 steps daily										
Sleep At Least 7 hours A Day										
Eat 50g of fiber daily										
Do daily self-accountability										
Effectively manage daily stress										
Lower daily expectations										
Maintain a healthy weight										
Keep your appointments and yearly physical										
Have Supportive relationships										
Eat five servings of vegetables and fruit daily										
Write 3 good things that happened to you every day										

Notes

Ardell DB(1999), Definition of wellness. Ardell Wellness Report,1999, 1-5.

Bains P (2020) Exercise to live longer. Allina Health

Be well BU; Learn practices that lead to better health and well-being. www.belmont.edu

Bussing A, Wirth AG, Reiser F, Zahn A, Humbroich K, Gerbersghagen K, Baumann K. Experience of gratitude, awe and beauty in life among patients with multiple sclerosis and psychiatric disorders. Health Qual Life outcomes.2014;12:63. https://pubmed.ncbi.nim.nih.gov/25102199/

CDC.gov; LDL and HDL Cholesterol: "Bad" and "Good" Cholesterol

Crouch M(2019) AARP

Chung I, (2005)Stress-Induced Atherosclerosis: Clinical Evidence and Possible Underlying Mechanism, Korean Circulation J 2005;35:101-105
Microsoft Word - 순2-1.doc (koreamed.org)

Debbie L Stoewen, (2017) Dimensions of Wellness. Can Vet J, 58(8): 861-862

Healing yourself with self-hypnosis, Frank Caprio, M.D. and joseph R Berger

Lin, J. and Epel, E.(2022) Stress and telomere shortening; Insights from cellular mechanisms. Ageing Res Rev.2022 Jan:73:101507. Published online 2021 Nov 1.doi 10.1016/j.arr.2021.101507

Mels Carbonell, Ph.D., How to solve the people puzzle. Uniquely You Resources, 2008.

Mills PJ, Redwine L, Wilson K, Pung MA, Chinh K, Greenberg BH, Lunde O, Maisel

A, Raisinghani A, Wood A, Chopra D. The Role of Gratitude in Spiritual Well-being in Asymptomatic Heart Failure Patients. Spiritual Clin Pract (Wash D C). 2015 Mar;2(1):5-17. doi: 10.1037/scp0000050. PMID: 26203459; PMCID: PMC4507265.

National Council on Aging(NCOA).(2023), Get the facts on Healthy Aging. www.ncoa.org

National Institutes of Health(.gov) https://www.ncbi.nih.gov.pmc
NSC(National Safety Council)2023: Injury Facts: Deaths by Demographics: Top 10 Preventable Injuries
https://injuryfacts.nsc.org//all-in

National Institute of Health(NIH) News.(2017), You're Never too Old. Keep active as you age.
https;//newsinhealth.nih.gov/special-issues/seniors/youre-never-too-old

Poljšak B, Milisav I. Clinical implications of cellular stress responses. Bosn J Basic Med Sci. 2012 May;12(2):122-6. doi:

10.17305/bjbms.2012.2510. PMID: 22642596; PMCID: PMC4362434

Robin G. Better Than Before: Mastering the Habits of Our Everyday Lives.Toronto, Ontario, Pengium Random House, Doubleday Canada, 2015.

Renna, M.E.(2021) A review and novel theoretical model of how negative emotions influence inflammation: The critical role of emotion regulation. Brain Behav Immun Health. 2021,Nov 25. Doi:10.1016/j.bbih.2021.100397 Retrieved from https://www.ncbi.nlm.nih.gov/pmc/articles/PMC8649080/

Sabot D, Lovegrove R, Stapleton P. The association between sleep quality and telomere length: A systematic literature review. Brain Behav Immun Health. 2023 Jan 9;28:100577. doi: 10.1016/j.bbih.2022.100577. PMID: 36691437; PMCID: PMC9860369.

Salleh MR. Life event, stress and illness. Malays J Med Sci. 2008 Oct;15(4):9-18. PMID: 22589633; PMCID: PMC3341916.

Shammas MA. Telomeres, lifestyle, cancer, and aging. Curr Opin Clin Nutr Metab Care. 2011 Jan;14(1):28-34. doi: 10.1097/MCO.0b013e32834121b1. PMID: 21102320; PMCID: PMC3370421.
Sorriento D, Di Vaia E, Iaccarino G. Physical Exercise: A Novel Tool to Protect Mitochondrial Health. Front Physiol. 2021 Apr 27;12:660068. doi: 10.3389/fphys.2021.660068. PMID: 33986694; PMCID: PMC8110831.

Smith, K. S., & Graybiel, A. M. (2016). Habit formation. *Dialogues in clinical neuroscience, 18*(1), 33–43. https://doi.org/10.31887/DCNS.2016.18.1/ksmith
Retrieved from Habit formation (nih.gov)

University of New Hamshire2023, Health & Wellness. www.unh.edu
https://www.unh.edu/health/intellectual wellness

University of Maryland:Dimensions of Wellness. Retrieved from (last accessed 2021) https://www.umaryland.edu/wellness/dimensions-of-wellness

Wood AM, Maltby J. Stewart N, Linley PA, Joseph S.(2008). A social-cognitive model of trait and state levels of gratitude. Emotion,2008;8(2):281-280. https://pubmed.ncbi.nim.nih.gov [Google Scholar]

WHO (2020)The top ten causes of death https://www.who.int/news-room/fact-sheets/details/the-top-10-causes-of-death

Yaribeygi H, Panahi Y, Sahraei H, Johnston TP, Sahebkar A. The impact of stress on body function: A review. EXCLI J. 2017 Jul 21;16:1057-1072. doi: 10.17179/excli2017-480. PMID: 28900385; PMCID: PMC5579396.

Resources

Here are additional resources that will help you live a healthier and longer life by consistently trying to be the best version of yourself in all aspects of your life. Did you know that you can become the best and happiest version of yourself every day irrespective of the situation or circumstance you may find yourself in?

www.compasswellnessinstitute.com
http://www.amazon.com/Dr.-Chio-Ugochukwu/e/B00JNFLPQQ
Join the compass club on Facebook
https://www.facebook.com/groups/17482 76835431116/

Other books by Dr. Chio Ugochukwu that will help you improve your health, eliminate stress and transform your life include;
The Compass Health Transformer: Your 72 Hour Blue Print For Healthy Living
In this book you will learn more about how doing the 72-hour food audit can help

you gain a better understanding of how you can improve your health through easy daily adjustments .....

21 Ways To Transform Your Health Without Medications

"...21 simple proven ways to reduce stress and improve your health and wellbeing without relying on medications. These are easy and effective ways you can use to turn your daily challenges into transformative opportunities for healthy living and daily happiness. You can start right away without spending a fortune!.."

<u>Get your own copy of 21 Ways To Transform Your Health Without Medications</u>

Overcoming Daily Stress: 21 Quick And Easy Ways To Stay Stress-Free In Your Daily Life

"...Are you tired of being stressed out everyday? Are you tired of feeling exhausted and overwhelmed in your daily activities? Are you fed up with communication issues in your relationship? Here are 21 quick and easy ways you can use to overcome daily stress and turn your daily challenges into opportunities for transformative abundant living. This book will help you gain a better understanding of your potential communication issues, daily 'stress points' and the steps you can take to overcome them…".

Get your own copy of Overcoming Daily Stress

The Secret To Daily happiness

"..Have you ever wondered why daily happiness has continued to elude you? Do you want to make sustainable daily happiness part of your life? By reading this book
you can find answers to these questions and many more on how to overcome the many obstacles and challenges that daily try to take away your inner peace and contentment…"

Get your own copy of The Secret To Happiness

15 Simple Ways to lower your blood pressure naturally after 40 without complicated diets

"……Don't spend your most productive years dealing with high blood pressure, medications and side effects. Stop worrying about whether you forgot to take your first medication or the second one. Take these simple steps to lower your blood pressure naturally and minimize your need for multiple medications. Did you know that high blood pressure can cause heart attacks, stroke, kidney failure, blindness and memory problems? Don't wait to find out! Take Action! ,,,,,"

Click Here for Your own copy of 15 Simple Ways To Reduce Blood Pressure....

Here is a book to help lose fat. If your main concern or focus is losing pounds you have accumulated as fat then get a copy of the book

---

"How To Lose 23 Pounds of Fat Without Torture Diets or Hard Exercise And keep it (The Compass Method).

"Are you fed up with trying to lose weight again and again with limited success? Are you tired of all the confusing new and expensive diets you have tried to follow every day with zero results? Do you want the health benefits of living with optimum weight without following complicated rules? Do you want to become more energetic and active again? Are you fed up with the wild ride of losing weight today and gaining it back tomorrow? Then read this book so that you will start using a comprehensive individualized weight loss strategy that will help you lose fat and keep it off, without going on torture diets or deadly strenuous exercises. You will learn to do this through the Compass Method that is based on a holistic approach to weight-loss, healthy living and personal transformation."

If prayer is something that appeals to you, you might be interested in the following next two books that incorporate prayers into our daily strive to become better and become more fulfilled:

Praying To Win: How To Get More Victories And Riches In Your Daily Life Through Spiritual Principles

"..You too can achieve your goals and dreams, through praying to win. You can do this by immersing yourself in the word of God and transforming the moments that make up your daily life through persistent adoration……. Above all, thank God every day, never give up and persistently continue praying to win…"

Get your own copy of Praying To Win

9 Best Ways To Eliminate Stress, Improve Your Health And thrive Without Limitations Through Prayers

Are tired of being knocked down by stress from your daily hassles? Are you tired of dealing with chronic illnesses associated with stress? Do you want to live a fun-filled daily life? Here are 9 of the best ways you can change your daily obstacles and challenges into opportunities to thrive without limitations through the power of prayers.

Too Young To Die

"A book about coping with grief and finding your way in life…"

9 Best Ways To Quit Smoking Without Becoming A Nervous Wreck And Gaining Weight

"..Here are 9 of the best ways to finally quit smoking without becoming a nervous wreck or gaining weight. If you have tried to quit smoking before, but failed or tried to quit but was overcome by anxiety or fear of becoming socially awkward or gaining weight, then read this book! This book was previously published as "The Compass Health Transformer Quit Smoking" but has been rewritten to include the transtheoretical model of change to help you get a better understanding of where you are in your journey or process of quitting smoking. The

9 best ways to quit smoking also includes a reminder of the different ways smoking can affect your health and body and the different individualized-changes you can make to your life-style to help you quit smoking on your own terms.

9 Best Ways To Deal With Negative People, Protect Your Health And Be Happy

"..Are you tired of being stressed out by encounters with negative people? Are you fed up with the impact of negative situations on your health and happiness? Would like you to find out ways to remain effective during negative situations and encounters with negative people? Do you know that chronic stress generated by negative encounters can damage your eyes, heart and brain? Do you know that chronic stress can directly damage your body cells? Here are 9 best ways you can protect your health from such negative situations so that you can continue to thrive and be happy..".

To order new or additional copies or ask questions, please visit:

http://www.amazon.com/Dr.-Chio-Ugochukwu/e/B00JNFLPQQ

Call or Text : 661 992 6436

Join the Compass club @

https://www.facebook.com/compassclub

About the Author

Dr. Chio Ugochukwu has always been interested in helping people live healthier, longer and more fulfilled lives through daily improvements in their health and wellness, and better self-care. He is focused on helping individuals and groups, use the compass method to develop their own compass blueprint or holistic process for healthy living, and self-mastery. Doing the 30-day challenge in this book will help you live longer by learning how to stay more consistently physically active, improve your self-accountability, sleep better, become more efficient at managing stress, and chronic conditions, and have more positive and supportive relationships.

Dr. Chio was inspired to develop the compass method for transformational living, through the challenges he has encountered in his journey of life, his practice of medicine, and his fascination with how the mind, the spirit and human experience influence the accomplishment of goals and the fulfillment of life, and his ancient heritage of Ozaa Akwusina (Warriors Never Stop).

He is the medical director of the Compass Wellness Institute and a consultant and specialist with interests in integrative medicine, ophthalmology, medical informatics, and public health. As an author, researcher, and consultant, he has peer reviewed publications on health and quality of life, and published more than 100 books and articles, on health and wellness, eye health, weight management, conflict management, stress management, effective communication, and integrative self-mastery.

To get some of Dr. Chio's books please visit:
https://www.amazon.com/author/chio